WELL
BEYOND
MEDICINE:
HEALTHY BY NATURE

Darrel O. Crain, D.C.

Coastal Sage Publishing
Alpine, California

The information and opinions expressed in this book are those of the author, and are true and complete to best of the author's knowledge. The information herein is not to be construed as medical or legal advice. The author and publisher are not responsible for any health effects or consequences resulting from the use of information in this book. Readers are urged to consult with the health professional of their choice concerning health matters. Indeed, seeking multiple opinions from different health practitioners is a sign of wisdom, and to be encouraged.

First published by Dog Ear Publishing
4010 W. 86th Street, Ste H
Indianapolis, IN 46268
www.dogearpublishing.net

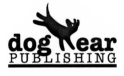

ISBN: 978-1-4575-1242-1

This book is printed on acid-free paper.

Printed in the United States of America

Dedication

I dedicate this book to all of you:

All the babies, young children, teens, and adults who have lost their lives or suffered devastating health damage caused by toxic exposure to medical interventions and other industrial poisons in the food, water, and the environment;

The many angels: The parents, siblings, husbands, wives, partners, and friends of millions of chronically ill and disabled people, whose daily lives must forever revolve around meeting the special needs of their health-compromised loved ones;

The personal freedom warriors: The thousands of people around the world who are working to establish the right of true informed consent, and the preservation and expansion of the right to choose or refuse all medical or other therapeutic interventions, without exception;

The natural health activists: The doctors, researchers, clinicians, teachers, and parents whose lives offer living proof that healing is an inside job that can be enhanced with sustainable, nontoxic support of the body's innate recuperative powers.

Contents

Preface vii

Acknowledgments...xi

Introduction..1

1. The Great Measles Misunderstanding 9
2. Childhood Vaccination: The Irrational Fear of Microbes.....15
3. Seven Laws for Saving Lives...20
4. Time to Split Up the FDA...24
5. Flu Shots For Pregnant Moms: Help or Harm? 29
6. Rewriting The Germ Theory 34
7. The Hygiene Hypothesis...38
8. Modifying Our Genetic Thinking..43
9. Washing Our Hands of Swine Flu Hysteria..........................48
10. Two Causes: Too Much, Too Little 58

11. Innate Healing and Nutritional Intervention........................62

12. The Wait-and-See Earache Prescription 69

13. Coughing Up the Facts on Whooping Cough......................73

14. Childhood Vaccination Against Sexually Transmitted
    Diseases: Protection For Whom? 79

15. Flu Season Again 90

16. The Doctor of the Future 98

17. Morning Sickness, Arbitrary Medical Rules,
    and Old Wives' Tales 103

18. Midwives Save Lives..107

19. Ultrasound During Pregnancy: Ultra-Unsound? 115

20. PreMedicine for PreProblems 120

21. Drugging Our Children..123

22. Coming Soon to a Child Near You: The War
    on Cholesterol 128

23. Breathing Easier Without Asthma Medication...................133

24. Sleep Makes the Grade 139

25. Getting Over Cold Medicine...143

26. Placebos, Real Drug Problems, and a Real Solution 147

27. One Flu Over the Cuckoo's Nest, or Dead Chickens
    Never Lie...152

28. FDA-Approved Viruses in our Victuals............................157

29. Drug Advertising Works 161

30. Asleep at the Wheel 165

31. The War on Breast Cancer 170

32. Fluoridation Nation 176

33. Killer Vitamins 184

34. Magnesium Magnificence 189

35. The War Against Vitamin D..194

36. Weighing in on Obesity and Inflammation.......................198

37. Taking Life One Day at a Time......................................202

38. Healthy Teeth, Healthy Spine, Healthy Heart 205

Bibliography 210
Index 213

Preface

Medical intervention, when appropriate, is remarkable, even miraculous, and justifiably expensive. The problem is that the vast majority of allopathic medical interventions are inappropriate, unnecessary, and even harmful—not to mention absurdly expensive. The late pediatrician and medical critic Robert S. Mendelsohn, M.D., estimated that as many as 90 percent of all medical interventions are neither appropriate nor necessary.

When an allopathic doctor finds clinical signs that stray from current customary standards, the question he or she automatically asks is, *What is wrong with you?* Allopathic medical doctors have been trained to presume that sick people have a broken or faulty internal regulatory system making mistakes, either because of genetic weakness or some disease process. Based on this assumption, pharmaceuticals are prescribed to override the body's innate regulatory levels.

But irregular clinical signs are often changes in physiology made by the body as it adapts to a stressful environment. Depending on the stressors in an individual's personal environment, such innate responses may be entirely appropriate.

For example, consider changes in blood pressure. A blood-pressure reading taken at rest that is found to exceed customary healthy values may be appropriate in an environment of stress. Imagine yourself in a stressful situation, say, being chased by a hungry lion. If your innate regulatory system did not fire up your adrenals and jack up your blood pressure so you could run faster than the wind, you would end up being the big cat's dinner. Later, when you are safely back home rubbing your sore muscles, your blood pressure goes back down.

Intelligent adaptation made by the body in response to environmental factors is called allostasis. An individual should not be presumed to have a pathology or disease based on abnormal clinical findings, because it is quite likely he or she suffers from a pathologically stressful environment; the body is merely matching physiological responses to its environment.

From an allostatic perspective then, the question the doctor should be asking is, *What is wrong with your environment?* Is the person eating a steady diet of fried fast food that makes his or her blood thick and sluggish? Higher blood pressure is needed to push that blood around in the body. Does the person seldom get any exercise, so the respiratory, blood, and lymph circulatory systems are inefficient, inflexible, and unresponsive? Higher blood pressure is needed to pump blood through such a congested body. Is the person living in a constant state of fear? Is he or she obese? Deficient in essential nutrients? High blood pressure can be a rational innate response to any number of negative environmental circumstances.

Working to eliminate the causes of adaptation is the hallmark of natural healing and health care. Many environmental stressors can be reduced or eliminated, allowing innate regulatory systems to reset to healthy levels, levels appropriate to less stress in the environment.

Allopathic medicine's "pill for every ill" strategy is deeply embedded in our culture, but more people every day understand that the pharmaceutical-centered disease-management approach is failing miserably. Parents who seek professional counseling for a child's behavioral or learning difficulties are still told their child has a disease of abnormal brain chemistry that will indefinitely require a prescription of daily narcotics. These same adults have watched their parents' health fade away on the medical merry-go-round with endless rounds of new pills, new problems, and no progress.

Learning to follow nature's laws for good health may not be easy, but those who ignore and disobey natural laws find that their health and healing has been arrested. Each person's biography becomes his or her biology. It is exciting to contemplate the day when young children know in their hearts from the earliest age that daily choices build future health. As generations of people make natural healing their first choice, watch the vast and powerful medical-industrial complex shrink to irrelevance and die a natural death.

In this book the reader will find unabashedly critical observations of a variety of health and medical topics that are intended to help lift the veil of false scientific authority that cloaks so much of what constitutes the practice of modern allopathic medicine here in the early 21st century. Skipping around in the book is just fine; the stories may be read in any order. I beg indulgence for the occasional note of irreverence that seems to have slipped into these pages.

Acknowledgments

Thanks to my supportive family: my wife, Nancy, my sons, John and Charlie, my mother, Isabel, my late father, Melvin, Cass, Greg, and Uncle Charlie. Special thanks to Linda Thompson and Cadi Goodnow. To Damon West, D.C., your ceaseless, mirthful merriment is greatly appreciated, as always.

Natural health practitioners stand on the shoulders of giants who blazed the trail before. I acknowledge here a few mentors whom I never personally met, yet whose words and work are an inspiration on the path of inquiry into all things natural.

B.J. Palmer, D.C., Ph.C., developer of the art and science of chiropractic wrote, *"We chiropractors work with the subtle substance of the soul. We release the imprisoned impulse, the tiny rivulet of force that emanates from the mind and flows over the nerves to the cells and stirs them into life. We deal with the magic power that transforms common food into living, loving, thinking clay; that robes the earth with beauty and hues and scents the flowers with the glory of the air."*

Max Gerson, M.D., demonstrated in clinical practice that the human body is innately capable of healing itself of even the most devastating and "incurable" health disorders.

Robert S. Mendelsohn, M.D., shared in his books the essential wisdom that the vast majority of medical interventions can be avoided by employing common sense, critical thinking, and simply allowing nature to take its course.

Bernard Rimland, Ph.D., fearlessly challenged the entire medical and scientific establishment on the causes of autism, and in the process brought hope and healing to families who had previously known only blame and despair.

Special acknowledgement must go to Ignaz Philip Semmelweis, the Hungarian physician who in the mid 1800s demonstrated scientifically that doctors were spreading infection and killing patients by not washing their hands. Semmelweis' reward for pioneering modern antiseptic procedures was rejection, ridicule, harassment, and a life in ruin. His legacy stands as a warning to all who dare to contradict and challenge the mighty medical status quo of the day.

Introduction

People accuse me of being an alarmist and tell me that things are not as bad as they seem. These people are correct on both counts. First, I am sounding as many alarm bells as I can possibly lay my hands on, and second, things are not as bad as they seem—they are far worse.

At some point in the last hundred years, the human condition became a medical condition. Every human physical and emotional challenge came to be viewed as a disease that requires treatment with drugs or surgical procedures, or both. The vast economic and political power of the medical industry has been used to create a pharmaceutical-dependent culture of medical crisis that is the basis of health care in the United States and other industrialized countries.

We are the original medication nation. We are number one in money spent per person on medical care. We are number one in consumption of pharmaceutical drugs. We are number one in using more vaccines and more drugs to fight more diseases than any other country in the whole wide world. All of which means we are the healthiest people on the planet, right? Painfully, we are not. Not even close.

International studies comparing the health of citizens in industrialized countries around the globe rank the United States at or near the bottom of every list comparing infant mortality, maternal mortality, life expectancy, and delivery of basic medical care. Prescription drugs have become a leading cause of premature death, exceeding the number of deaths from either illicit drug use or traffic fatalities. Vaccines are now widely associated with multiple autoimmune and neurodevelopmental disorders. Multiple epidemics of chronic illness continue spinning out of control.

It has come to this: Human beings are an endangered species. A confluence of environmental, public health, and medical factors threatens our health today and the health of future generations.

Rising Living Standards

Over the course of the past century and a half, massive reductions in mortality from infectious disease were realized in modern societies the world over. The discovery of vitamins and other essential nutrients in combination with the advent of indoor plumbing, modern sanitation, and antiseptic medical care resulted in the precipitous drop in the death rate from infectious disease well before antibiotics were available or mass vaccination programs established.

Nevertheless, our public health officials' heads are stuck in the 19th century, prior to the rise in living standards, at a time when infectious disease represented the major health threat to our citizens. Accordingly, precious public resources are squandered on scientifically unsupported, clinically irrelevant, and physiologically toxic public health campaigns such as the annual flu shot pageant.

A profound misunderstanding of the vital interdependence among humans and microbes has spawned decades of medical antibiotic misuse and abuse. This has accelerated the evolution of super bacteria resistant to every last antibiotic in existence, and millions of people now suffer intractable digestive disorders due to the loss of friendly, health-producing gut flora following antibiotic therapy.

Life as an Enduring Medical Condition

First, consider pregnancy and birth. From time immemorial birthing was a natural process patiently nurtured by midwives and doulas, but it has been commandeered over the past century and a half by medical men who turned it into big business. Pregnancy was transformed into

2

a disease state requiring ongoing medical intervention, while the birthing process was reinvented as a dangerous medical procedure requiring hospitalization and a standard sequence of medical interventions that often disrupts and effectively halts the natural birthing process. All too frequently this leads to emergency Cesarean section surgery to deliver the baby, which is major abdominal surgery that poses additional risks of maternal complications, infection, and longer recovery. Artifacts of the customary epidural and labor-inducing agents given during medically directed birthing spike fevers and provoke breathing distress in many newborns, which mean transfers to the neonatal intensive care unit and the strong likelihood of additional drug interventions—all of which place the child's immediate and long-term health at greater risk.

Next, take the vaccines. Health authorities are convinced that humans are incapable of mounting proper immune responses to wild bacteria and viruses encountered naturally in the environment. This presumption is the apparent basis for government-sponsored mass vaccination programs that promote cradle-to-grave inoculations and booster shots to "fool" the immune system into producing antibodies against an ever-growing list of microbes.

Pediatric medicine's so-called well-baby checks are the final stage in our nation's assembly-line vaccine-delivery system. One size fits all, y'all! The busy, growing vaccine schedule recommended by our federal government (which is literally in the business of selling vaccines) is traditionally rubber-stamped as mandatory by elected state governments (whose treasuries are rewarded—using federal taxpayer money—for complying with federal vaccine recommendations). Hundreds of new vaccines are on the way.

Growing older was once a natural passage of aging, but it has been transformed into a perilous journey that is survivable only with continuous medical interventions and considerable luck. When a senior citizen such as my mother shows up for her insurance-required annual medical checkup, the medical staff seem unable to fathom that an octogenarian can just say no to prescription drugs and live a healthy and remarkably active life.

Industrial Food

It took fewer than 100 years for industrial farming to take over virtually all food production. We are simultaneously choking on industrial food with its toxic herbicide and pesticide residues while starving from its lack of vital nutrients.

Factory-farming practices raise animals under horrendous conditions and produce animal-based foods that are highly contaminated with antibiotics, synthetic growth hormones, bacteria, viruses, and filth. Rather than force industrial food producers to clean up their act, government agencies have approved measures to "sanitize" food, such as irradiation.

Genetically modified (GM) foods are full of novel proteins that are suspected of causing disruption to immune function. These are being foisted one after another upon an unsuspecting public because manufacturers are not required by the U.S. Food and Drug Administration to label GM foods. We are witness to an unprecedented epidemic of food hypersensitivities and life-threatening allergic reactions across all age groups and ethnic populations, all across the nation, even as the FDA continues to throw all caution (and GM pollen) to the wind and to allow more and more genetically modified food genies out of the bottle.

In synch with the shift to Big Food production has been the cultural shift to fast-food consumption. Such meals consist of "foodlike substances" that satisfy the taste buds with high levels of low-quality fats, high-fructose corn syrup, highly refined carbohydrates, artificial sweeteners and coloring, and the ever-present neuroexcitatory chemical additives such as MSG. But a steady diet of these products starves the body of vital nutrients, while paradoxically triggering massive weight gain and the resultant loss of physical fitness and health. People who regularly eat this fare become progressively overweight and disabled with the symptoms of chronic inflammatory degenerative disease, a condition some call Sedentary Death Syndrome.

Environmental Toxins

The scope of cumulative environmental neurotoxic exposure is difficult to comprehend because the sources literally surround us. Mercury and radioactive particles are in the air, mercury and PCBs (polychlorinated biphenyls) are in the water, and numerous other toxic industrial chemicals are in both the air and the water, as well as in household cleaning products, personal care products, and food packaging. Toxic industrial waste residues are purposely added to public water supplies in the form of water fluoridation, a practice based on the scientifically unsupported claim that doing so improves dental health.

Added together with the plague of "normal" background air pollution that is emblematic of modern industrialized societies, all this industrial pollution exacts a heavy toll on human health.

Emotional toxicity is another chemical toxicity, only this one is created within the body. Fear stimulates the fight-or-flight response, flooding the whole body with stress hormones, which prevents the body from winding down into a state of homeostatic rest and cellular repair, a perfect storm for chronic illness.

Vaccine Toxins

Mass vaccination programs are a major source of neural and immune toxicity, despite ardent denials by the medical community. These programs repeatedly expose people—especially our children—to aluminum, mercury compounds, carcinogenic and neurotoxic chemicals, and immune-disrupting foreign proteins. As a principle of biology, any living system with any exposure whatsoever to these substances is adversely affected to some extent.

Unfortunately, vaccination stimulates only the adaptive response of the human immune system and not the innate response. At best this provokes a temporary expression of antibodies, and it requires repeated reinoculation just to maintain circulating antibodies.

Unbelievably, no study has ever monitored the effects of receiving multiple vaccines all at once, nor has any study ever compared the health of vaccinated versus unvaccinated children. Studies of the effects of exposure to the mercury component of vaccines (thimerosal) have compared only children with varying levels of exposure to the mercury compound; no comparison has been made to children with zero exposure.

Vaccination represents only one of many neurotoxic environmental assaults on the developing brain and nerve system of a child, albeit a very potent and oft-repeated one. The scientific literature provides broad evidence of immunological and neurological impairment in children, directly resulting from exposure to the reactive ingredients found in vaccines.

A subpopulation of children appears to be biologically impaired in the ability to properly clear toxins from their bodies. This results in cellular damage, mitochondrial dysfunction, systemic dysfunction, and resultant severe physical, developmental, and behavioral health problems. Children diagnosed with Autistic Spectrum Disorder, Pervasive Developmental Disorder, Childhood Disintegrative Disorder, and various other

5

named conditions share a variety of health disorders. These include chronic inflammatory bowel problems, food allergies and sensitivities, sensory and auditory processing difficulties, frequent viral infections, recurring ear infections, symptoms associated with encephalopathy, and motor skill deficits, as well as the classic social interaction and communication challenges.

Outbreaks of childhood infectious disease in fully vaccinated populations are now commonplace, suggesting that the term "vaccine-preventable diseases" is entirely erroneous and needs to be changed to the more accurate "vaccine-*alterable* diseases." The tragic irony is that for many children, far from preventing targeted infections, vaccination induces chronic immune system dysfunction and severe gut dysbiosis, which seriously depresses the child's innate expression of good health. Once we are able to move past the archaic notion that we must medically prevent infection, we can get on with the real work of building strong people who have strong immune systems for life.

Pharma-based Disease Management

Medical offices today are filled with people suffering from chronic illness, illnesses which typically arise from nutritional deficiencies and toxicity in the body due to unhealthy life habits. Unfortunately, standard allopathic treatment is pretty much limited to pharmaceuticals and/or surgery. But drugs depress healthy function in the kidneys and other organs and use up vital nutrients. This stimulates ever-greater systemic inflammatory responses and further depletes stored nutrients. The result is the suppression of normal, healthy physiology in the cells, tissue, and organs throughout the body every day of the year, year after year.

After decades of pharmacological disease management and the inevitable downward spiral of health, the tragic finale is typically a heroic, futile, medical battle against death due to cataclysmic organ failure in the final few weeks and days of life. One drastic intervention after another is piled on, and the outrageously high cost of all the end-stage medical drama frequently devours the entire life savings of individuals, couples, and families.

Saying No to the Drug Industry

We have tremendous work to do. Anyone who seeks to create naturally good health is up against the culture of perpetual medical crisis

6

that has been conjured by the largest and most powerful cartel of corporations in the history of humankind. The wall separating the pharmaceutical industry from public health and regulatory agencies has disintegrated, leaving the corporate foxes guarding the proverbial henhouse.

The broadcast media's dependency on Big Pharma advertising revenues inevitably censors and corrupts fair and accurate reporting about problems with the medical status quo, trivializes scientifically based drugless healing disciplines, and levels attacks against inexpensive, time-honored, natural healing traditions.

Professional medical associations and their drug company sponsors are actively at work in states across the nation attempting to dismantle parental rights of informed consent and the freedom to choose or refuse medical interventions. Big Pharma recently flexed its political muscle in California and shepherded through the legislature a new law that thwarts parental authority entirely, allowing the marketing of controversial vaccines against sexually transmitted diseases directly to 12-year-old girls and boys.

We are witness to the criminalization of refusal of medical intervention. Armed agents of state and federal governments are enforcing compliance with medical authority. Parents have been arrested and their children taken away into "protective custody" for refusal to follow doctor's orders to give their children chemotherapy, psychiatric drugs, and vaccines.

Even so, the information age continues to shine an ever-brighter light on the once-hidden limitations and dangers of standard allopathic medicine, hastening the day when medical authority will be crushed under the weight of its own massive contradictions.

Healthy by Nature

Healing is an inside job. The body's powerful innate forces that produce good health need the proper resources to express their greatest potential. Health care interventions that support innate healing tend to be sustainable, noninvasive, low-risk, and long-term. Interventions that address both sides of the health coin—deficiency and toxicity—offer the greatest potential for healing and lasting health. Unfortunately, doctors whose allopathic training compels them to understand every health disorder as a disease or genetic defect are prevented from witnessing the remarkable recuperative powers of the human body once it is properly nourished, allowed to clear itself of toxicity, and maintained in proper biomechanical motion.

Which brings up the question, is your allopathic doctor saving you or killing you? Will the surgical procedure being proposed or the drug being prescribed help or harm? It is up to you to decide. It has fallen to the individual health consumer to sort out which intervention is helpful and which one is harmful.

As a society, we must respect and encourage personal health freedom. The freedom to choose or refuse any and all health care interventions, medical or otherwise, without coercion, is an inalienable human right of every individual and every parent. This fundamental freedom is not to be legislated away or in any way compromised by an elected or appointed official, nor by any governmental agency under any circumstances. Fully informed consent in the absence of coercion was guaranteed for all humanity for all time in 1947 in Nuremburg and set down in the Nuremburg Code.

The quest to create good health for you and your loved ones is not only rewarding, it builds character. You get to stand up to any knuckleheaded doctors in your life and fire them straightaway if they do not agree to support you in your unique and personal journey on the path of natural health and healing. After all, they work for you, not the other way around. Settle for nothing less than what your gut instinct tells you is best for you and your family.

Consider adopting a simple rule of thumb that has the potential to help you and yours live healthier, more vital lives: *Educate before you vaccinate or medicate.* The benefits of avoiding unnecessary medical interventions far outweigh the risks of offending family members and medical doctors.

The Great Measles Misunderstanding

Mankind has survived all catastrophes.
It will also survive modern medicine.

Gerhard Kocher

Before the advent of the measles vaccine, a dozen or so cases of measles would have been considered, well, too measly to make the headlines. That is because we all got the measles when we were kids. In fact, the Centers for Disease Control and Prevention (CDC) considers everyone born before 1957 to be immune to the measles.

"Before a vaccine was available, infection with measles virus was nearly universal during childhood with more than 90 percent of persons immune by age 15 years," according to the CDC's Pink Book.

We baby boomers apparently were the last generation whose doctors, and, therefore, parents, accepted the measles as just one more annoying rite of passage of childhood that also happened to prime the immune system and provide lifelong immunity.

Medical texts prior to the advent of the vaccine described measles as a benign, self-limiting childhood infectious disease that posed little risk to the average well-nourished child. All that changed about 40 years ago when health authorities decreed the need to eradicate the measles, and so began The Great Measles Massacre.

A recent measles outbreak in Southern California provides an opportunity to review how effective the overall strategy of measles eradication has been so far.

First of all, measles-related deaths had already declined over 90 percent from the early 1900s by the time the measles vaccine came on the scene. The combination of steadily improving standards of living, better nutrition, antiseptic medical care, and effective sanitation achieved this remarkable advance in public health in the "prevaccine" era.

One of the first measles vaccines tried out on a large scale was the inactivated, or "killed," measles vaccine (KMV). The CDC's Pink Book reports that "an estimated 600,000 to 900,000 persons" in the United States were injected with KMV from 1963 to 1967, before it was finally withdrawn.

The incredibly imprecise record of how many people received the shot is a bit unsettling, but what is truly disturbing is how such a harmful and ineffective vaccine got approved and recommended in the first place. "KMV sensitized the recipient to measles virus antigens without providing protection," the Pink Book tells us. After exposure to natural measles, vast numbers of people vaccinated with KMV contracted atypical measles, an autoimmune disorder consisting of very high fevers, unusual rashes, pneumonia, and pleural edema.

Devastating the health of so many people in the war against measles cannot be called collateral damage; it is friendly fire. Friendly fire is a wartime phrase that describes inadvertently firing upon one's own soldiers or other friendly forces in the attempt to engage enemy forces, especially when it results in injury or death.

The really big campaign against measles began with the live virus vaccine, which arrived in 1971 as a component of the three-virus MMR shot (measles, mumps, rubella). The public was assured that this vaccine was different, it was going to be safe, and it would provide lifetime immunity. Alas, these rosy predictions were apparently based on nothing more than optimism.

"An outbreak of measles occurred in a high school with a documented vaccination level of 98 per cent," reported the *American Journal of Public Health* in April 1987.

"We conclude that outbreaks of measles can occur in secondary schools, even when more than 99 percent of the students have been vaccinated and more than 95 percent are immune," reported the *New England Journal of Medicine* in March 1987.

An interesting side note is that the word "immune" once meant that a person was protected from a disease due to the action of his or her immune system. Nowadays people are said to be immune just because they have vaccine-induced antibodies circulating in their bloodstream, even if they readily get the disease from which they are supposedly protected.

By the mid-1990s, substantial vaccine failure with the MMR shot prompted our health leaders to declare a booster MMR shot necessary for everyone. Once again, we were promised this would confer lifetime immunity. Presumably, since no actual lifetime data were available at the time, this was yet another prediction made using FDA-approved crystal-ball technology.

Today, the number of reported measles cases is down considerably, and we are told that this statistic by itself means we have successfully massacred the measles. Unfortunately, such a one-dimensional analysis fails to tell the whole story. Not all is well with the MMR.

Before widespread vaccination against measles, young babies were not at risk of measles because they acquired immunity through the mother's blood. Adults were not at risk because we acquired lifelong immunity following a bout with measles as a child. Both these groups are now susceptible to measles infection, and both age groups have greater risk of severe disease and complications. This is described as an "unintended outcome" of measles vaccination.

And there is another unforeseen problem. "The vaccination-induced measles virus antibodies decline in the absence of natural booster infections. It is important to follow how long the protection achieved by the present vaccine program will last after elimination of indigenous measles," reported the journal *Vaccine* in December 1998.

This raises an important question: What will happen as we eventually succeed in replacing wild measles with vaccine-induced measles? David Levy, M.D., of Montefiore Medical Center in New York created a computer model to answer that question, and reported that "despite short-term success in eliminating the disease, long-range projections demonstrate that the proportion of susceptibles in the year 2050 may be greater than in the pre-vaccine era."

In other words, he projects that the net result of vaccinating the entire population for 90 years will be more people getting the measles than we started with, except that infection will be spread throughout those age groups who are at greater risk of serious illness.

Currently, whenever there is an "outbreak" of measles (defined by the CDC as at least two infections from the same source), health officials leap into action. First and foremost, parents are told to drop everything and make sure their child gets a booster shot. Does giving the booster shot during an outbreak actually help? We don't know for sure, since few studies have ever asked that question.

At least one such investigation was carried out during a measles outbreak in a highly vaccinated secondary school population, as reported in the *Canadian Medical Association Journal* in November 1996. The authors concluded, "Administration of a second dose of vaccine during the outbreak was not protective."

Are there any other strategies out there that can protect the health of children infected with measles? Yes. Supplementing with vitamin A has repeatedly been shown in clinical trials all around the globe to be effective at reducing the severity of measles infection, as well as slashing the death rate following infection.

This suggests that our health leaders should be promoting vitamin A as a first line of defense to protect children in this country, especially since measles deaths in the United States have always been clustered in impoverished, malnourished populations.

British vaccine expert witness Jayne Donegan, M.D., is a parent who has spent years researching vaccines. She has concluded, "I vaccinated both my children with the MMR jab, but this was before I started my research into the problems associated with it. Knowing what I know now, I would not vaccinate my children and run the risk of them getting diabetes, asthma, eczema, becoming more susceptible to meningitis and ending up chronically disabled."

If you have been waiting for the FDA to step in and investigate the many safety issues that have cropped up in the history of MMR and the other vaccines, you'll have to take a number and get in line. It seems that all three FDA employees who actually check on food and drug safety issues are busy closing down a small company that produces canned cherries—they were found to be printing unproven health claims on their labels about the benefits of eating cherries.

"The FDA will not tolerate unsubstantiated health claims that may mislead consumers," said Margaret O'K. Glavin, associate commissioner for regulatory affairs. "The FDA will pursue necessary legal action to make sure companies and their executives manufacture and distribute safe, truthfully labeled products to consumers," according to an FDA press release.

This impressive new declaration by the FDA that it will begin demanding truthful labeling is a breath of fresh air. It may help us move toward actual informed consent in medicine, especially in the mass vaccination programs. And, since we are on the subject of measles, I propose the following new label for the MMR vaccine vial, just to make sure consumers know exactly what has been substantiated about the vaccine so far:

"This product contains substances known by the U.S. Government to cause harm to human beings, including cancer, autoimmune diseases, nuerodevelopmental disorders, and allergies. Genetically susceptible individuals injected with this vaccine are known to suffer enterocolitis, nerve system dysfunction, and autism spectrum disorder. Antibodies in the bloodstream provoked by the vaccine do not necessarily confer protection from measles infection. Paradoxically, in order for any vaccine-induced immunity to work at all, the vaccinated person must come in contact with the natural, wild measles virus from time to time. The maker of this product cannot be prosecuted for any disability or death caused by the vaccine to you, your babies, or your children. If something does go wrong and your kid gets seriously sick, good luck with suing the government because the likelihood that you will receive compensation is approximately zero."

At last count there were about seventeen jillion government- and vaccine-industry-funded articles published in journals that claimed to disprove any possible link between vaccination and autism. With each new report, the medical community has harrumphed loudly and declared that this piece of work, finally, will be the last nail in the austism/vaccine coffin, the definitive study that will lay to rest forever any foolish questions of vaccine safety.

Barbara Loe Fisher, cofounder of the National Vaccine Information Center, notes that no amount of reporting on cherry-picked data mined from old medical records in various foreign countries does any good to erase our current epidemic of profoundly sick children here in the United States.

"Using pencils and calculators to dismiss causal associations between vaccines and chronic diseases is easier than having to look at real live patients or study what happens to their blood, urine, eyes, brain, colons, etc., after vaccination."

Has the time come to rename the whole measles eradication enterprise as *The Great Measles Misunderstanding*? The history of vaccination against measles is replete with tragic health-damaging errors, unanticipated negative outcomes, a misplaced faith that mass vaccination is the unquestioned master plan, and in all likelihood the whole program will ultimately make measles more of a problem than it was in the prevaccine era.

The tragic collective denial by our health leaders that manufactured, government-recommended viral and bacterial vaccines are devastating the health of thousands of children a year is nothing short of criminal. The medical industry and public health authorities have been tinkering with the natural order of microbial exposure and infection within our population for decades now. The results are in: The biological integrity of our children is being fatally compromised.

Next time you read an editorial that castigates parents for choosing to avoid vaccination, keep in mind that one day soon the same writer may instead be writing words of gratitude to the vaccine refusers. It turns out that those who are volunteering to skip the vaccine are keeping the pool of circulating wild measles virus alive and well, to the benefit of everyone.

Childhood Vaccination:
The Irrational Fear of Microbes

The greatest threat of childhood diseases lies in the dangerous and ineffectual efforts made to prevent them through mass immunization.

Robert Mendelsohn, M.D.

Have you ever noticed that young children seem programmed to seek out and contact every existing microbe in their surroundings? On playgrounds around the world, little ones walk up and lick each other's faces even though they are complete strangers, and wander from one spot to another sampling the dirt, as a chef might sample her soup.

Ah, yes, microbes. When I was in grade school, measles, chicken pox, and mumps were considered no big deal. In fact, as soon as any kid in the neighborhood showed any telltale signs of infection, moms used to arrange impromptu parties just to make sure all us kids got exposed at the same time.

There would be contests taking turns with the same whistle to see who could blow the loudest note, followed by blowing up balloons and letting the air out and then swapping balloons with other kids to blow them up again. Our moms knew how to make saliva mixing fun.

The time-honored tradition of accepting each childhood infection as a rite of passage has waned over the years, overtaken by a much different agenda, heavily promoted by public-health leaders and pharmaceutical companies. The goal nowadays is pretty much the opposite of my childhood experience. Today's parents must labor under the medical mandate to vaccinate against more and more childhood infectious diseases, with the apparent goal of avoiding natural infection altogether. The prevailing policy is prevention at all costs because the medical community believes that the benefits of vaccination outweigh the risks of infection.

Medical science is determined to conquer every single germ—one shot and one child at a time. If you want to say goodbye to fevers, skin blisters, rashes, sore throats, pustules, and all that other yucky stuff that used to be part and parcel of growing up, all your kid needs today, we are told, is a very, very long list of shots.

A recent count of the recommended shots for girls is about 156 vaccine antigens in 45 shots, and for boys, about 144 vaccine antigens in 42 separate shots. Of course, next year another shot, perhaps two, will probably be added to the list along with, undoubtedly, another couple of booster shots. Oh, and don't forget about giving your kids their two flu shots every year. And so on. I am told that at least one hundred additional vaccines are in the developmental stage, and the federal government seems to rubber-stamp every single shot that comes along and add it to the list.

Unfortunately, parents who wonder aloud why so many vaccines are necessary these days may quickly be branded as anti-vaccine. Patients tell me stories about being "fired" by their pediatrician after asking why a particular vaccine was necessary for their child, and then asking the doctor to just skip that vaccine. This can be very puzzling to parents who are just trying to make sure they are doing what is best for the health of their child.

If your pediatrician is okay with answering a few questions about vaccines, try asking this one: "Are we sure that vaccinated kids are healthier than unvaccinated kids?" You can be fairly certain that he or she will answer, "Oh yes, the benefits far outweigh the risks." After this reassurance is made, ask the doctor to name one scientific study that has ever addressed this question, just one. The doctor will be unable to name such a study because none has ever been undertaken. Ever.

In the unlikely event that your pediatrician answers honestly by saying, "Well, I was taught in medical school that vaccinated children are healthier than unvaccinated children, but I have never personally seen the science," tell the doctor you want to see the science yourself before giving your kid any shots. In the highly unlikely event that the doctor actually does try to find the studies for you, discovers there are none, and then reports back to you, ask the following question: "Isn't it time we answer that most basic of questions before we even think about giving one more shot to one more child, considering that each shot adds another syringe full of neurotoxic and carcinogenic chemicals, neurotoxic metals, and immunogenic foreign protein fragments—agents of immune dysfunction—into our kids?"

As the priority in public health evolved to become the prevention of childhood infectious diseases, a lower incidence of infection with a given microbe was accepted as proof that mass vaccination was the very best thing for our children's health. But is it as simple as all that? The answer is no.

For example, not only are measles, mumps, and whooping cough outbreaks quite common among highly vaccinated populations, but infection with measles now occurs in much younger and much older populations, for whom the illness is often far more dangerous.

And then there is chicken pox, the mild, self-limiting illness once revered in many cultures as a visit from a goddess. As the chicken pox vaccine was being licensed for widespread use, critics of the plan predicted that one result would be a massive shingles epidemic in the older population, causing excruciating pain and chronic, unrelenting suffering in our senior citizens. This prediction was based on the projected loss of wild varicella virus circulating in the community, whose presence is needed to periodically rekindle immunity through exposure, thereby preventing shingles outbreaks.

Tragically, the critics were correct. Senior citizens in the United States are now suffering an unprecedented shingles epidemic. Was it just a coincidence that a new vaccine was immediately rolled out to fight shingles and "protect" older people from varicella? In case you are wondering what they put in the new shot, here it is: the same toxic cocktail found in the children's chicken pox vaccine, only with fourteen times more viral material.

Regarding the chicken pox vaccine for children, Edward Yazbak, M.D., commented, "We replaced a simple self-limited disease with a nasty, painful and chronic one. When will we learn that it is not wise to try to fool Mother Nature? We think we have a solution to a problem only to find out that our solution is the problem."

Evidence continues to pile up that the heavy vaccine schedule in the United States may be responsible for our scandalously high infant mortality rate. The *Journal of Human and Experimental Toxicology* in May 2011 published a study comparing vaccine schedules and infant mortality rates among thirty-four countries. The authors concluded that their findings "demonstrate a counter-intuitive relationship: nations that require more vaccine doses tend to have higher infant mortality."

Enthusiasm for mass vaccination, based on a severely limited understanding of how repeated vaccine exposure affects our children, and a complete disregard for the cumulative toxic burden it creates, is causing serious and widespread collateral health damage—especially in those children whose bodies have a diminished physiological ability to clear toxins.

Medical leaders would have us believe that the entire health profession is united in its support of mass vaccination programs. Thankfully, increasing numbers of medical doctors and research scientists are speaking out against the wildly unscientific nature of our one-size-fits-all, jam-packed vaccination schedule. Unfortunately, many of these brave souls have found themselves attacked, ridiculed, and even blacklisted by their peers, licensing bodies, and professional organizations for asking any questions about vaccines.

An honest appraisal of the whole mass vaccination process—from deciding which vaccines to develop to the shocking inadequacy of vaccine safety trials and subsequent government licensing and mandating—must conclude that the entire effort is fraught with gross financial conflicts of interest and blatant disregard for authentic scientific investigation.

Meanwhile, parents around the world are horrified to see neurodevelopmental disorders and chronic diseases devouring the good health of their children, robbing them of the potential for normal, productive lives. Alarmingly, these tragic epidemics are peculiar to modern industrialized countries whose populations are subject to the highest rates of childhood vaccination. Public health leaders are at a loss to explain the cause of these epidemics, yet we are constantly and vehemently reassured that vaccines cannot possibly be blamed for any of this.

Rita Hoffman of the Vaccine Information Awareness Network has asked a key question, "What would be the general state of health today if 200 years ago medicine had taken the path of discovering the keys to promoting a strong, unadulterated immune system in conjunction with increased nutrition, vitamin and mineral supplementation along with better sanitation?" Indeed, many parents are following that path on their own, despite their pediatricians' and family doctors' irrational and unscientific fear of microbes.

Seven Laws for Saving Lives

Natural forces within us are the true healers of disease.

Hippocrates

It was in the midst of the tragic Spanish flu pandemic of 1917-19. People were dying right and left from secondary bacterial infections that overwhelmed their weakened immune systems after contracting the influenza virus. The medical men of the day had no antibiotics to pull out of their little black bags. Many remedies were tried, including calomel, also known as mercurous chloride. Some historians have speculated that the use of this mercury-containing compound for the sick may have actually cost the lives of more than a few patients.

But there were three groups of doctors healing the stricken with no drugs whatsoever: chiropractors, osteopaths, and homeopaths. These doctors were in great demand because they were losing very few patients to the dreaded flu. In fact, the legendary ability of chiropractors and osteopaths to keep their patients alive and well during the epidemic is largely responsible for the subsequent licensure of those two health disciplines in several states, and public health records of the era show that homeopaths treated many thousands of patients during the pandemic and achieved survival statistics that could only be envied by allopathic medical practitioners.

Chiropractors were examining and adjusting their patients' spines with the intention of restoring normal spinal nerve function and nerve system communication. Osteopaths were performing spinal manipulation with the intention of enhancing lymph flow. Each of these two disciplines of so-called physical medicine was working with the spine to restore and enhance immune function in the body. Hippocrates himself, the father of medicine, spoke of this vital concept more than 2,000 years earlier when he wrote, "Get knowledge of the spine, for this is the requisite for many diseases."

As you can imagine, the already powerful and wealthy medical establishment at the time was none too happy with this kind of nonmedical claptrap. Organized medicine could neither understand nor control these pesky healing arts that required no drugs and so set about trying to belittle and destroy them with labels of unscientific quackery and cultism.

As Dr. Benjamin Rush, Declaration of Independence signatory wrote, "Unless we put medical freedom into the Constitution, the time will come when medicine will organize itself into an undercover dictatorship...."

Indeed, organized medicine has been busy these many years, deliberately and systematically working to destroy not just chiropractic, but also midwifery, naturopathy, herbalism, and homeopathy.

The long history of the American Medical Association's (AMA) fight against nonmedical healing arts has seemingly never been about improving the health of patients. "The history of the AMA is resplendent with a long, illustrious, and unbroken tradition of trying to do away with its competition. In each case, the AMA appears to have been motivated more by the desire to monopolize the medical market than by wanting to help people or protect them from frauds. How else, for example, can we explain the organization's war on chiropractic?" wrote John Robbins in his book *Reclaiming our Health*.

Chiropractic is still regarded as an orphan of the health care field because of its historic, stubborn refusal to get involved with drugs. Osteopathy, on the other hand, which had always been a completely drugless and bloodless healing art, was ultimately seduced and swallowed up by organized medicine to join the world of drugs, surgery and insurance coverage.

Alas, mighty modern medicine, ruler of virtually every aspect of the health care realm, is a modern-day emperor who wears no clothes. I say this because of the naked truth of this paradox: Medical intervention is a leading cause of premature and unnecessary death in this country. Imagine several jumbo jets crashing every single day all year long with no survivors, and you can begin to imagine the enormous level of collateral carnage caused collectively by medical intervention, no matter how well intentioned each single act might be.

Where is the outcry? Where are the investigations into why hundreds of thousands of people need to die unintentionally each year from FDA-approved medications? Where are the emergency federal programs charged with reducing this incomprehensible number of preventable annual deaths? Why do medical doctors think me rude when I ask such questions at parties?

Never one to miss an opportunity to breach social etiquette for the chance to save a few lives, I offer here my *Seven Laws for Saving Lives*, a set of rules written to help people take control of their own health and avoid the substantial health risks associated with even the most innocent sounding drug therapy. Obviously, these laws are my own opinion—the expression of which is protected under the first amendment of the Constitution—and are not to be construed as medical advice.

There is one piece of advice, however, that I offer freely and without hesitation to everyone: Seek a second, third, and even fourth opinion from the qualified health professional of your choice. Doing so is neither cowardice nor folly, it is a sign of wisdom. And for heaven's sake, do not limit yourself to consulting only those health practitioners under contract with your medical insurance company.

The first law: *Above all is respect for the right of every individual to medical freedom, individual choice, and true informed consent.*

The second law: *Use watchful waiting unless faced with an emergency. Nature requires time to heal. Symptoms are evidence that healing is taking place. Suppressing symptoms interferes with natural healing processes and may promote chronic disease.*

The third law: *Engage and feed the body's powerful healing forces with live foods, pure water, and daily physical and mental exercise. The key to healing is often found in correcting deficiencies and eliminating toxicities in the body.*

The fourth law: *Follow these cautionary ABCs if you plan to take any drug, whether prescription or over the counter: (a) a family history of adverse drug reactions; (b) any health condition that may be adversely affected by the drug; (c) any herbs, supplements, or other drugs also being taken that may interact harmfully.*

The fifth law: *Seek the lowest dose and the shortest possible duration of time if drugs are taken.*

The sixth law: *Trust in the body's miraculous innate healing potential, and never lose hope, nor take away hope from another.*

The seventh law: *Live a lifestyle of wellness. Profound and unexpected health benefits are commonly experienced, and the prevention of chronic illness later in life is quite possible.*

"Nature alone cures and what nursing has to do is put the patient in the best condition for Nature to act upon him," wrote Florence Nightingale, considered the founder of modern nursing.

Government and industry leaders in the health field have an opportunity to heed Nightingale's time-tested advice, especially as they anticipate and fear new flu pandemics each year. Common sense and history suggest that the best way to prepare for viral outbreaks and enhance the health of our nation is to seek out those healing disciplines and natural health strategies that are nontoxic and sustainable, and have proven to help people survive and thrive, no matter what virus is circulating in the community.

Time to Split Up the FDA

All bad precedents began as justifiable measures.

Julius Caesar

Will it ever be safe to eat salad greens again? From where I stood in the produce section of the supermarket, I could see the headlines screaming from the news rack by the checkout counter: CONTAMINATED PRODUCE! PEOPLE SICKENED! I glanced suspiciously at the onions on my left. Were they tainted? I leaned over and cautiously sniffed the spinach. Had rogue pigs gotten loose and run rampant through the spinach patch, spreading E. coli in every direction, just moments before the greens were picked, packed, and shipped?

The poor U.S. Food and Drug Administration (FDA) has certainly been overwhelmed with problems of food and drug safety lately. Perhaps we are asking too much of those erstwhile commissioners to keep track of both our food and our drugs. After all, how can we expect them to effectively police the vegetable farms of America when they are already up to their ears writing black-box warning labels for already approved drugs that are unaccountably killing and disabling thousands of people? There just isn't enough time at the end of the day to think about food, beyond grabbing a quick hormone-tainted, antibiotic-laden hamburger with GMO fries and an artificially sweetened soda on the way home to get a few hours of sleep.

One problem is that medical schools do not really equip doctors to understand the profound importance of food and nutrition. Big Pharma's powerful economic influence over medical school curriculum and culture perpetuates a narrow focus on pharmaceutical therapies to the exclusion of any understanding about the principles of natural healing. These powerful economic behemoths prefer that no one finds out too much about adequate diets, healthy lifestyles, and living with the body in balance and structural alignment because it could ruin them financially.

Medical practitioners do, however, emerge from medical school enthusiastically poised to scribble prescriptions for dangerous drugs all day long. That is why we need to free up more time for the FDA research doctors to improvise fast-track approval for the newest and scariest drugs and bizarre vaccines.

Each new drug requires much creativity and imagination to invent and name a new disease to go along with it, not to mention planning the jillion-dollar marketing schemes with the cunning ads that send people in droves to beg their doctors to prescribe that new pharmaceutical as soon as it comes down the pike. The average person has no idea how much time all this takes, what with flying back and forth to drug-company conferences at five-star hotels in exotic locations around the globe, each one with mandatory rounds of golf and lavish four-course banquet dinners, followed by much drinking and flirting with scantily clad cocktail waitresses.

Back in the day when the only drug question on the table was whether aspirin should be taken on an empty stomach or with meals, it probably made sense that the responsibilities of keeping watch over food and drugs should be combined, but things are quite different today.

Many people, even many working inside the FDA, mistakenly believe that the essence of a food or nutrient is no different than the essence of a drug. In an effort to provide food for thought and help FDA researchers digest the difference between the two, I hereby provide the following definition of food, as articulated by the online American Heritage Dictionary: "Material, usually of plant or animal origin, that contains or consists of essential body nutrients, such as carbohydrates, fats, proteins, vitamins, or minerals, and is ingested and assimilated by an organism to produce energy, stimulate growth, and maintain life."

From the same dictionary we learn the definition of a drug: "A substance used in the diagnosis, treatment, or prevention of a disease or as a component of a medication. A chemical substance, such as a narcotic or hallucinogen, that affects the central nervous system, causing changes in behavior and often addiction."

Obviously, there are stark and fundamental differences between food and drugs. In recognition of the fact that eating nutritious foods in proper proportions can often eliminate the need for any drugs whatsoever, a conflict of interest clearly exists within the hallowed halls of the FDA. I believe it is high time to split up the FDA into two separate agencies.

The drug part of the agency we will call the Drug and Disease Administration, or the DDA. Medical doctors can head up this one because they have been formally trained to see every aspect of the human experience as a medical condition requiring prescription drugs for treatment, a second drug to treat the side effects of the first one, the third and fourth drug for the second, and so on up to a dozen or more drugs per person.

The food agency will be called the Food and Natural Healing Administration, or the FNHA. Wellness doctors and nutrition experts can run this one because of their propensity for viewing human health challenges as the result of nutritional, emotional, structural, spiritual, and lifestyle imbalances. By dividing up the FDA house in this way, everyone will be working on projects they like and know best, and everyone will be happy.

Don't get me wrong, though, there will still be ample opportunity for collaboration between the two distinct, new agencies. For example, it makes no clinical sense to stick with the outmoded practice of comparing drug effects only to placebo effects. (As a side note, remember back in the good old days when they were using actual placebos in the drug trials, instead of doctored up pills that produce side effects similar to the unpleasantness caused by the actual drugs being tested? Or the vaccine placebos which contain the same toxic metals and chemicals as the vaccines being tested? But I digress.)

The time has come for us to move well beyond simple drug/placebo testing. If it is health we are looking for, let us perform high-quality scientific research that compares health outcomes among (a) drugs, (b) placebos, and (c) restoring health on the cellular level using nutrition, exercise, and energy restoration. With two separate agencies steadfastly representing the best ideas in their respective fields, it will finally be possible to level the playing field and understand which protocols get the best results.

When the research starts pouring in and the data tallied, many folks will be amazed at the results that can be achieved by the foodies and natural healers. Wild claims that hundreds of billions of dollars can be saved each year, not to mention saving hundreds of thousands of lives in the process, can finally be scrutinized in a strictly scientific fashion and may just be proven correct.

If that is the case, drug companies will no doubt find they need to hire more spin doctors to massage, manipulate and mangle the data before they can profitably market their drugs. Not to worry though, the pharmaceutical industry has proven enormously resilient when forced to put a positive spin on catastrophic news, superseded only by its skill at spreading fear in the public mind about diseases that are either as rare as a winning lottery ticket or fictional disorders invented by public relations hacks. (But Restless Legs Syndrome? Come on guys, that one was so lame. Any good clinician could have told you it isn't a disease at all, simply a clinical red flag for magnesium deficiency.)

Yes, things will definitely be different once we have a pro-food agency that does not push drugs. Before long, producers of high-quality organic fruits, vegetables, nutrition supplements, and herbs may find they have ample scientific evidence to go head to head in the marketplace against anticancer drug therapies that do nothing to stop the cancer but cost as much as buying a new house. No longer will there be armed FDA storm troopers raiding producers of raw milk and other natural products and shutting them down because they had the audacity to cite published scientific literature indicating measurable health benefits available to users of their products.

We might even discover that children whose parents just say no to more than 50 vaccinations before they even show up for their first day in school are actually healthier than those who get stuck as if they were human pincushions. At any rate, for the first time in history, the health of vaccinated children will finally be compared to that of unvaccinated children. Armed with this information, people will finally have a chance to analyze scientifically verifiable results for themselves, allowing them to make truly informed choices about the health of their own children.

I know what you are thinking: Who in the heck has the money to pay for another federal agency in Washington, D.C.? No problem. The

FDA's funding pretty much all flows from the deep pockets of Big Pharma already. No need to mess with that revenue stream. In fact, once we remove food from the crowded plate of the new Drug and Disease Administration, drugs will begin flying out of the drug pipelines faster than you can say, "Stock split on Wall Street!"

Ah, but what about funding for the new Food and Natural Healing Administration? The solution to that is simple also, but requires a bit of political will. We need to tap into the very source of sickness, the undisputed king of chronic illness in North America: television advertising. Look at it this way, the public owns the public airwaves and we also own the broadband spectrum. We have a legitimate right to charge higher rent to mega-corporations for the privilege of coming into our living rooms to brainwash us.

I realize that the drug companies are the ones with the largest advertising outlays, so unfortunately, their industry will be the one most affected by this modest new tax. I am not too worried about it though, if you take just a moment to look at Big Pharma's unfathomably enormous profit margins, you will notice they can easily afford it. Besides, you may recall that some of the most profitable blockbuster drugs in history were discovered and developed at American universities using taxpayer money. Once the real work was done, the patents were simply handed over to drug makers to go out and make another killing—in some cases, literally. Here is a chance for the boys from down on the pharma to show some gratitude and pay back a few billions in kind.

But time is of the essence. For the public's protection we need to separate food and nutrition issues from the pharmaceutical cartel's stranglehold as soon as possible. For starters, the farmers of this country urgently need a government agency to help them figure out how to wash the produce before it goes on the trucks, not to mention the urgent need to get the drug executives out of the debate on vitamin safety. Otherwise, natural foods and vitamins will become contraband and I will get arrested for felony possession of a slab of raw-milk cheddar cheese on my sandwich and a bottle of vitamin C crystals in my briefcase.

Flu Shots for Pregnant Moms:
Help or Harm?

*Once we accept something as "good," we often persist in doing it
even when the result is clearly bad, while telling ourselves
that we just haven't done enough of it.*

Dave Kopel

How is it possible that the wealthiest nation on the planet has an infant mortality rate higher than just about every other industrialized country in the world? And what can we do about it? Help is finally on the way for solving this dilemma, or so I thought when I first noticed the newspaper headline announcing new recommendations for pregnant moms from the Centers for Disease Control (CDC).

Before reading the article, I leaned back in my chair and began making a mental checklist of possible ways to help pregnant moms birth healthier babies.

I thought of the requirement by the Food and Drug Administration (FDA) a decade ago to add folic acid, a B vitamin, to food. This simple step has achieved an impressive reduction in the number of babies born with spina bifida and other central nervous system defects.

Perhaps the CDC would be offering more advice about nutrition? The impact could be huge if America's pregnant moms ate a more balanced and healthy diet. Poor diet is associated with low birth weight and premature delivery, both of which are linked to a higher infant death rate.

I thought about the importance of exercise during pregnancy. Had the CDC embraced this low-tech, nontoxic intervention to increase the chances for full-term deliveries and, therefore, healthier babies?

I thought about the fact that using antibiotics and over-the-counter pain medication during pregnancy causes a much greater risk that the baby will develop asthma and other atopic diseases. Was the CDC putting out a warning to doctors and pregnant moms to avoid antibiotics if at all possible?

Then it struck me: Maybe someone in the CDC had been talking to the midwives about the neurology and biomechanics of pregnancy, and why babies may remain in undesirable breech or posterior positions, often resulting in cesarean section deliveries. Could it be that the CDC was going to recommend that the neuro-biomechanics of the pelvis be balanced with a short course of spinal corrective care by a qualified chiropractor employing the Webster technique?

I was feeling giddy with thoughts of all these excellent possibilities and how sharing these ideas with all the pregnant moms in America could make a major contribution to healthier babies, and…that's when the cat jumped into my lap, startling me out of my daydream and snapping my thoughts back to reality.

"The truth will set you free," said Mal Pancoast, "but first it will piss you off." A variation on that same theme works perfectly here: "If you aren't outraged, you are not paying attention."

I looked down at the newspaper and read what the CDC now had in mind for pregnant women: Through its committee called the Advisory Committee on Immunization Practice (ACIP), the CDC had just recommended flu shots in all three trimesters of pregnancy.

Flu shots. That's right, flu shots. This was puzzling news indeed. Weren't pregnant women as recently as a year ago told to avoid vaccination out of concern for neurological harm to the mother and the baby? How come pregnant moms were suddenly the target of massive, aggressive campaigns by public-health authorities, HMOs, and doctors to get their flu shots?

"The CDC advises pregnant women to get flu shots either with or without thimerosal," according to the National Institutes of Health Web site. Thimerosal is the ethylmercury preservative used in flu shots. I wondered if any CDC officials had bothered to read the fine print on Elli Lilly's Material Safety Data Sheet for thimerosal: "Exposure to mercury in utero and in children may cause mild to severe mental retardation and mild to severe motor coordination impairment."

I looked for evidence that the CDC had conducted or discovered new studies showing that flu shots are safe for pregnant women and their babies. None were mentioned. How about the other ingredients in the flu shot besides mercury that are also neurotoxic in even the tiniest amounts? Had they successfully removed the aluminum phosphate, the polysorbate 80, and the formalin, a formaldehyde derivative? Nope. Was there new evidence that the flu vaccine actually reduces the incidence of influenza-like illness, making it an important contribution for reducing infant mortality? No. In fact, there was no scientific evidence presented to support the new guidelines.

I had no recollection that the flu had ever even appeared on a list of risk factors during pregnancy for either moms or babies. The CDC's own records show only a few hundred documented deaths from the flu across the entire country each year, and these occur mostly in the elderly and immune compromised. The official government citation that 36,000 people die each year from the flu is apparently calculated by flu experts using special flu math, in which the confirmed number of actual influenza-related deaths is multiplied by a factor of at least 120.

As I read further on in the article, the words of power that are used to justify every questionable medical intervention on the planet jumped out of the newspaper and into my face: The Benefits Outweigh the Risks. This phrase is so powerful that it trumps every conceivable objection to any controversial medical intervention, and ruthlessly silences the mightiest of opposing ideas. These five words carry the full and terrible weight of unquestionable and unimpeachable medical authority, and if you disagree, well, you're a nut job.

What *are* the benefits, I wondered? What *are* the risks? I sought answers to these questions in one of the few non-pharmaceutical-industry-funded research papers I could find on influenza vaccines, published in the Summer 2006 *Journal of the Association of American Physicians and Surgeons*, authored by F. Edward Yazbak, M.D., and David Ayoub, M.D.

First, the benefits: "There is no convincing evidence of the effectiveness of influenza vaccination during this critical period."

Okay then, how about the risks? "No studies have adequately assessed the risk of influenza vaccination during pregnancy and animal safety testing is lacking."

What about the mercury in the shot? "Thimerosal, a mercury-based preservative present in most inactivated formulations of the vaccine, has been implicated in human neurodevelopmental disorders…including autism, and a broad range of animal and experimental reproductive toxicities, including teratogenicity, mutagenicity and fetal death."

Teratogenicity, according to Dorland's Medical Dictionary, means "the development of abnormal structures in an embryo resulting in a severely deformed fetus." The meaning of the term mutagenicity is "causes mutation."

In the conclusion of the article the authors state, "The ACIP policy recommendation of routinely administering influenza vaccine during pregnancy is ill advised, unsupported by current scientific literature and should be withdrawn. Use of thimerosal during pregnancy should be contraindicated." Contraindicated means it's a really bad idea and it should be stopped.

"Trivalent influenza virus vaccination elicits a measurable inflammatory response among pregnant women," according to the journal *Vaccine* November 2011. Measurably increases inflammation? This should raise a huge red flag for the strategy of influenza vaccination during pregnancy, since inflammation is associated with preeclampsia and preterm birth. But the reaction from flu shot promoters is predictable—all together now: "The benefits far outweigh the risks."

I have absolute faith that the average person can draw sensible conclusions about his or her own health, but only if he or she is given all the facts. This is definitely not happening. In the realm of public-health endeavors such as the annual push for flu shots, serious concerns, concerns based on sound biological principles regarding toxicity, as well as negative outcomes that have been discussed in peer-reviewed, published medical journals, are routinely denied, dismissed, and trampled in the fearful flu commotion each year.

I would not presume to know what is best for anyone else regarding his or her own health, or whether or not the flu shot is for you. My efforts are devoted to the preservation of medical freedom and the realization of true informed consent. I also like to point out the one option that is available to all but seldom gets discussed during flu season: It may be wise to explore the avoidance of all medical interventions whenever possible, especially if you are a pregnant mom, considering our country's unforgivably high infant mortality rate, plus the fact that medical error and unintended complications from standard medical interventions comprise one of the top killers in the country each year, right up there with heart disease, cancer, and stroke. I'm just saying...

Just then the cat jumped out of my lap and onto the windowsill, taking an interest in a bird just outside the window. At that moment I recalled words of wisdom from a fellow named Steve Plog that fit perfectly with my thoughts on medical authorities giving flu shots to pregnant moms: "According to the World Health Organization, America is the 37th healthiest nation in the world. Basically, the American Medical Association's team is in 37th place. When was the last time you took the word of a 37th place team as gospel?"

Rewriting The Germ Theory

*It is time to lay to rest the notion that germs jump into
people and cause diseases.*

Emanuel Cheraskin, M.D.

I received some startling news the other day that left me totally
bugged. "You're standing there telling me that 90 percent of the
total number of cells I carry around in my body are microbes?" I
gasped.

"Get over yourself," my friend the microbe expert said offhandedly,
surprised I didn't know this already. "We humans are only 10 percent
human cells and the rest teeming, thriving microorganisms along for a
symbiotic ride."

She pulled out a 2004 report from the American Academy of Microbi-
ology and read to me, "Microbes enable efficient digestion in our guts,
synthesize essential nutrients, and maintain benign or even beneficial

relationships with the body's organs. The presence of these organisms influences our physical and mental health."

I had to sit down immediately. That is, "we" had to sit down, my microbes and I. Why had I never understood or even heard about this before? What is the significance that so many more cells in our bodies are microbial than human? Who or what controls the other 90 percent of me that is not me? When the fundamental importance of germs to human health is fully appreciated in the field of health care, won't there be a massive revolution?

At the very least, I thought, it was high time to rewrite The Germ Theory.

Of course, there always have been a few "bugs" in the germ theory of disease that have prevented the theory from graduating from the hypothesis category into a full-blown principle of medical science. First off, if germs alone really did cause disease, none of us would be left standing here to discuss the theory's finer points. There is obviously something else at work here, perhaps the ability of us humans as hosts to maintain resistance and develop immunity.

Louis Pasteur himself apparently found it necessary to fudge the results of major experiments he carried out just to make the germ theory work, according to historian Gerald Geison in his book *The Private Science of Louis Pasteur*, published in 1995. Geison was one of the very first scholars given the chance to study Pasteur's personal notes following the Pasteur family's long-delayed release of the research. I imagine the new portrait of Pasteur that emerged in Geison's book did not go over too well with the French people, who have erected beautiful statues and named venerable public institutions after him.

Pasteur reportedly worked hard to garner credit for developing the germ theory during his lifetime, even though scientists had already been kicking the idea around for a hundred years or so before he showed up. As an old man, though, Pasteur is said to have dropped the entire germ theory and sided with his contemporary, Claude Bernard. Bernard was the doctor who once gathered a group of colleagues around him and quaffed a glass of water teeming with cholera bacteria, proclaiming, "The terrain is everything; the germ is nothing!" By this act Bernard staked his health on the belief that a "germ" requires the right kind of "soil," namely, diseased tissue, to mount any kind of infection that results in illness.

Many germ theory enthusiasts find the idea intolerable that Pasteur might have abandoned his pet germ theory in old age and sided with Bernard. They dismiss his 180-degree change of heart as the incoherent ravings of a sick and dying man. Others believe Pasteur was very sound of mind at the time he changed his mind and deserves credit for publicly declaring that the available evidence of the day supported an entirely different story.

At the very least though, the germ theory rescued us from the Evil Spirits Theory, which was the dominant theory of disease before blame was reassigned to germs. This is now regarded as a giant step forward for science. That is because the cures for casting out evil spirits required the use of harsh treatments that ended up killing significant numbers of people needlessly. I am told this in no way resembles modern medicine's incessant war against microbes, whose harsh treatments end up killing staggering numbers of patients unintentionally each and every day.

Considering that microorganisms help us digest our food, create vital nutrients, and protect us from opportunistic infections, is it any wonder that antibiotics and vaccines are linked to so many terrible health disorders, complications, and chronic diseases, since their effect is to kill, baby, kill?

If microbes could talk, they would launch a public-health campaign and declare, "Poison to one is poison to all!" If the human body were ruled by democracy, the microbes in our bodies would hold an election, and the germ majority would vote to prevent pharmaceutical attack whenever and wherever possible.

Which brings us back to the task at hand, the rewriting of the Germ Theory of Disease. Since germs are such a big part of who we are, it follows that our good health depends on the good health of our resident microbes. We need a brand new manifesto for creating good health that centers on making our microbes feel safe, welcome, and right at home. In short, we need to make peace with our microbes, love our microbes, and ask our microbes what they want for dinner.

The new theory could be called the Germ Theory of Life instead of the Germ Theory of Disease. The transition period will require that all of us reach deep down inside and exercise patience and understanding to help reform well-meaning but misguided germ haters and killers. Medical practitioners especially will face enormous challenges and difficulties at first, because they have been trained to the core to maintain a constant state of war against germs and to kill every germ in sight, not to mention the invisible ones. Luckily, people in the health field tend to have good hearts, and they will naturally excel in the new system once they make the transition to being germ lovers. Indeed, many health professionals have already seen the writing on the wall and have taken up the new slogan—I Love My Germs!—with gusto.

But the armies of professionals working for the Big Pharma Drug Cartel will not stand down easily. The very foundation of the pharmaceutical industry was built upon suppressing and killing microbes. Without the germ theory, the greatest and most powerful economic force in the entire history of humankind will find it increasingly difficult to justify perpetual germ warfare and germ genocide. We can expect Big Pharma to cling to the germ theory as tenaciously as the Catholic Church once clung to the belief that Earth was at the center of the universe. Heads may roll before the transition to loving our germs is complete.

If we step back and gaze at the bigger picture of public-health history, we see that scientific advancement lurches and zigzags down the road of progress like a drunken sailor, as theories come and go, and old dogmas and their promoters die off. Cries of Death to the bugs! will slowly fade as we learn to nurture our bugs and raise the healthiest bugs possible.

Humans are but a small part of the stream of nature. Our good health ultimately depends on the health of our environment, which is a complex, interdependent community of life, and each one of us constitutes our own internal environment or ecosystem.

Not surprisingly, the habits we need to learn to ensure the happiness of our microbial cells are identical to the things we need to do to ensure the health of our human cells. These include the usual suspects: eat well, think well, exercise well, rest well, love well, and be well.

Thankfully, at this point in history we are relatively free to choose good health and create a healthy lifestyle. Embracing the new Germ Theory of Life does not require a prescription, a physician, or anyone's permission.

The Hygiene Hypothesis

Sickness is the vengeance of nature for the violation of her laws.
Charles Simmons

"Your prescription is ready Mrs. Jones, fresh intestinal whip-worm eggs straight from the pig."

This type of medicine, called helminthic therapy, may sound rather unorthodox, but scientists are testing this unusual treatment on human patients for a surprising variety of ailments, from asthma and inflammatory bowel disease to multiple sclerosis.

"Take two tablespoons of dirt and call me in the morning." That may also sound like a bit of a stretch, but then again, it is possible that mud pies may one day be squeezed into the five food groups if the hygiene hypothesis continues gaining ground. The time has come to get down and dirty in the good fight for good health.

The hygiene hypothesis holds that many health disorders are the unintended consequence of ultracleanliness in modern societies, and the remedy for some of these disorders may be renewed exposure to pathogens and parasites.

The germ theory, however, which still holds sway with modern allopathic medicine, maintains that we get sick because of something we "catch." Sickness in this view results from some germ we ate, inhaled, or were otherwise exposed to that invades our body. Those of us brought up on the germ theory have been trained to constantly wage war on germs. Kill! Disinfect! Sanitize! And when you finish with all that, go wash your hands.

American industry has gleefully led the charge in the war on germs. At last count there were approximately 700 quintillion products that murder, massacre, mutilate, and otherwise destroy germs, including antibacterial soaps, lotions, cleansers, sprays, tissues, hand wipes, toys, mattresses, socks, and even computer screens.

Ironically, much has been written in the medical literature about the dangers of going crazy killing germs with antibacterial soaps and the like. It appears that the potent chemicals in these products actually contribute to the evolution of new, scary, and currently untreatable microbial infections rather than reduce infection. Oh, and by the way, some of these killer chemicals are known to kill human cells pretty effectively, too.

The hygiene hypothesis may sound like the name of a junior high home economics course, but it encompasses a completely different way of thinking about health by taking the germ theory and turning it on its head. In this view, germs are not something we should fear; rather, we should invite our neighborhood germs over for a friendly chat and breathe them right up our collective noses.

Proponents of the hygiene hypothesis argue that early exposure to a wide variety of microbes is a good thing, permitting a growing child's immune system to develop and grow, learning appropriate immune responses, thereby building up immune response "muscle."

While the germ theory leads down a white, sanitized, sterilized, fumigated, and bleached hospital hallway, the hygiene hypothesis decisively turns the cart off the road and heads down an old dirt path surrounded by living creatures.

Researchers have long noted and described in the medical literature an important difference among children who attend daycare at a very young age, live with many brothers and sisters, have lots of pets in the house, or live on a farm. Compared to children raised in a more anti-septic environment, kids with greater exposure to microbes of all kinds appear to develop less asthma, hay fever, allergies, eczema, and other atopic diseases. Interestingly, many autoimmune diseases at epidemic levels in industrialized countries are rare or entirely absent in rural, less-developed countries.

But a lack of exposure to a wide variety of environmental microbes is only half the problem. In simple terms, there are two legs to our immune system. The first, our innate immune response, or Th1 response, can be thought of as the low-key neighborhood cop who provides protection without making a big fuss. The Th1 cop takes care of the ordinary, everyday identification, tagging and dismantling of microbes, and then makes sure to create memory cells that enable rapid recognition and disposal of the menacing microbials in the future. However, if your friendly Th1 cop never encounters microbes as you grow up, he or she never learns how to properly do his or her job.

Insufficient stimulation of the Th1 leg of our immune system also results in too much stimulation for the second leg of our immune system, the Th2, or adaptive, response. The Th2 response can be thought of as the combined forces of the FBI, fire department, CIA, NSA, SWAT team, National Guard, United States Marines, Naval Reserves, and Coast Guard, all responding at once. You can just imagine the juris-dictional disputes and contradictory strategies that occur in this situa-tion. The Th2 response is the proinflammatory response, which explains why Th2 cells are found to be active in many autoimmune dis-eases. Atopic disorders are characterized by immune responses that are inappropriate and completely out of proportion to the actual threat at hand.

Standard medical practices are known to provoke the Th2 response. Exposure at a young age to antibiotics, antipyretics (fever-lowering drugs), and vaccines have all been observed to raise the risk of asthma and the other atopic disorders in comparison with the health of chil-dren who do not receive those medications.

One Swedish study describing this phenomenon was published in the journal *Lancet* May 1999. The researchers found that children whose parents avoided giving antibiotics and vaccinations as much as possible suffered fewer atopic diseases than did the children in the study who routinely received such medical interventions.

The list of disorders that can be iatrogenic, meaning they are trig-gered by doctor-prescribed medications, includes autoimmune responses such as multiple sclerosis, rheumatoid arthritis, inflammatory bowel disease, and even type I diabetes.

"Half the modern drugs could well be thrown out the window, except that the birds might eat them," commented Martin Fischer.

In our zeal to kill every possible germ with a pharmaceutical preparation, we have apparently succeeded in suppressing the robust expression of innate immune responses to normal childhood illness and set the stage for chronic inflammatory processes in adulthood.

A healthy immune system should be expected to periodically whip up a robust healing crisis, it is simply doing its job of defending against invasive microbial infections. And yes, the symptoms are bound to be uncomfortable. However, the inconvenience and suffering that comes with periodic immune workouts yields benefits that last a lifetime—namely, an immune system with a strong innate response, permanent immune memory, and the absence of chronic inflammation as one gets older.

The hygiene hypothesis leads to some intriguing, even shocking, questions. Do you suppose nature intended all those kids at day care to be infected with various cold viruses, spike the occasional fever, rest in bed for a few days, and then go back for more? Is it possible that Mother Nature herself wants us all to have a bout with the chicken pox, measles, and, yes, even the mumps and whooping cough while we're still young?

In return for allowing nature to pump up our innate immune muscle we are given permanent, noninflammatory immunity, as well as an enhanced likelihood of appropriate immune responses for the rest of our lives.

How much healing actually requires medical expertise? I have personally observed the scraped knee of a three-year-old toddler heal just as quickly and thoroughly as the knee of a Harvard-trained medical doctor with multiple board-certified specialties. It comes as no surprise to me that nature's plans for our immune system manage to avoid the numerous pitfalls created unintentionally through human effort. It appears that we may be carrying the "cleanliness is next to godliness" habit too far and may need to cut back on well-intentioned medical interventions.

The hygiene hypothesis forces us to ask another important question that does not even occur to mainstream medicinal practitioners: Which is preferable, expression or suppression?

Repeated vaccinations are intended to suppress infections. The trouble is that outbreaks of mumps and other "vaccine-preventable" childhood illnesses occur in highly vaccinated adult populations with regularity. The perpetual solution of mainstream medicine is to add more booster shots. Each shot stimulates more proinflammatory Th2 immune responses while inhibiting the innate Th1 response, setting the stage for chronic illness.

What does expression mean? Pediatrician Lawrence B. Palevsky, M.D., notes that "children need to be allowed to experience symptoms of acute illness in order for their bodies to appropriately cleanse the wastes and toxins from their systems, and so they can go forward in their lives toward greater optimal health and wellness." In other words, kids have to get sick to be well.

The medical literature provides substantial evidence suggesting that many standard medical practices, based as they are on the prevention and suppression of infections and symptoms, are associated with high rates of chronic, inflammatory health disorders. Maybe we should be spending less time trying to fool Mother Nature and more time learning to trust our miraculous, innate recuperative abilities. Maybe we should worry less about which germs our kids "catch" and instead encourage them to spend more time running around and playing outdoors, acting like kids and getting dirty.

The compost bin of medical history overflows with once-revered medical practices whose supposed benefits crumbled to dust long before their use was discontinued. History also shows that outmoded medical practices live on until they are finally buried, along with the practitioners who championed them.

Who is to say whether many of today's drugs and shots won't be replaced by worms and dirt? After all, doesn't everything eventually return to dirt, dust, and ashes? As the old saying goes, *Eat right, exercise regularly, die anyway.*

Modifying Our Genetic Thinking

Natural healing is not about avoiding doctors.
It is about not needing to go to doctors.

Andrew Saul, Ph.D.

Big Pharma is currently funneling billions of dollars into genetic research to fight disease. The goal is to isolate specific genes that cause obesity, cancer, diabetes, heart disease, and many other disorders and then disable, kill, or remove the offending gene, thereby preventing the genetic expression of that particular condition or disease.

This strategy is based on a long-held belief that genes control the health of the body. Theoretically, this requires the human genome—the full set of human genetic instructions—to contain 100,000 genes or more, one for each protein the body makes, and quite a few others to turn the expression of genes on and off. This theory is known as genetic determinism, and some call it the central dogma of modern allopathic medicine.

The Human Genome Project was launched in 1990 in an effort to move medical science closer to the dream of gene-based medicine, with the ambitious goal of mapping and cataloging all 100,000-plus genes. However, several years into the project, a surprising development emerged. The scientists in charge reduced their estimates and said they now expected to find only 30,000 to 35,000 genes. With the project nearing completion in 2004, the estimate was again revised downward to only 20,000 to 25,000 protein-coding genes inside the nucleus of human cells. The scientists noted in a press release at the time that it was "a surprisingly low number for our species," about the same number of genes found in the DNA of the average rodent.

"Now that the Human Genome Project has toppled the one-gene-for-one-protein concept, our current theories of how life works have to be scrapped. No longer is it possible to believe the genetic engineers can, with relative ease, fix all our biological dilemmas. There are simply not enough genes to account for the complexity of human life or of human disease," declares world-renown cell biologist Bruce Lipton, Ph.D., in his book *The Biology of Belief*.

Dr. Lipton writes that "the notion that genes control biology has been so frequently repeated for such a long period of time that scientists have forgotten it is a hypothesis, not a truth….We want to believe that genetic engineers are the new medical magicians who can cure diseases and while they're at it create more Einsteins and Mozarts as well."

Despite compelling evidence to the contrary, genetic engineers and medical researchers cling to their belief they can eventually cure disease in this way. Even the pernicious and widespread problem of serious adverse reactions to prescription drugs is being blamed on "genetic variants."

"The dogma is so fundamental to modern biology it is essentially written in stone, the equivalent of science's Ten Commandments. The dogma, also referred to as 'The Primacy of DNA,' is a fixture of every scientific text," writes Lipton.

I found myself hoping Dr. Lipton was wrong about outdated dogma living on in our children's textbooks. Perhaps the textbooks in classrooms today had been successfully updated with the latest science, and biology students were now learning that human genes play a much different role in maintaining the health of the body than we have always presumed, an entirely passive role. Hoping for the best, my son and I cracked open his new high school biology book. We flipped to the chapter on cell life, and there in black and white was the old dogma staring us right in the face, "The nucleus manages all cellular functions." Rats! It turned out Lipton was correct; an entire generation of potential future scientists is still being educated with outdated, fundamentally flawed scientific theory.

Merriam-Webster's online dictionary defines dogma as "something held as an established opinion." Also, "a doctrine or body of doctrines concerning faith or morals formally stated and authoritatively proclaimed by a church."

Which reminds me of Copernicus and Galileo, two of the greatest intuitive scientists and scholars in human history. They desired to share with humanity their understanding that Earth does not lie at the center of the universe. Unfortunately for them, the ancient, skulking dogma chained to the massive gate fronting the Catholic Church growled and howled when he heard about this new blasphemy. The highest holy men of the Church knew they had to keep the dogma happy or risk losing their moral and political sway over the common people, so they busied themselves throwing the dogma a bone. The errant scholars Copernicus and Galileo were promptly hauled in and given a stern lecture about the facts of life according to the Catholic Church: Earth always has been, and always will be, at the center of the universe.

You may recall that these events occurred in the early 1600s, so, unfortunately, the meetings were not captured on video and posted on YouTube, as might be the case today. Even so, I imagine the session with Copernicus went something like this: "Your holinesses, my observations through the telescope and my careful scientific calculations have led me to conclude that Earth is an insignificant planet, cast in a permanent orbit around our sun with a bunch of other planets; the sun is only a minor star in the far reaches of a minor galaxy, and we have no idea where the heck the center of the universe is—but we do know with a fair amount of certainty that Earth is nowhere near the center."

The wise religious leaders showed decisive leadership by immediately clapping their hands over their ears and yelling loudly, "La-la-la! Cannot hear you!" And with black robes flapping, they all scurried out of the room, slamming the heavy wooden door behind them. After calming themselves with some thoughtful draughts of holy wine followed by prayerful meditation, the holy men returned to confront Copernicus. "You have two choices," they sharply intoned, "either recant this ungodly blaspheme that humans and Earth are not at the center of the universe or else spend the rest of your miserable days under house arrest!"

History shows that scientific progress has frequently been arrested by the dogma of religious, political, and business leaders of the day, with the information typically held hostage as long as those leaders remained in power. Luckily for modern-day astronauts, the old Catholic Church leaders had died off by the time humans were planning to send a spaceship to the moon, and scientists were at liberty to declare that the earth does, in fact, orbit the sun.

Which brings us back to the central dogma of medicine. In order for medicine to progress, we need leaders who can let go of the old dogma and accept the new scientific understanding. Genes are expressed by the human body/mind as adaptations to stimuli (or lack thereof) in the environment from moment to moment. How about redirecting those billions of dollars of research into the elements of the human experience already known to modify genetic expression? A partial list of environmental influences includes emotion, nutrition, exercise (or lack thereof), and stressful experiences that trigger the stress response and flood the body with stress hormones, such as physical and emotional trauma.

Children diagnosed with autism spectrum disorder provide a dramatic example of how we may alter environmental factors to overcome serious health disorders. Partial and even complete recoveries for thousands of these children from their autistic behavior has been achieved using functional medicine or biomedical protocols that address underlying problems of inflammatory gastrointestinal dysfunction, metal nuerotoxicity, and hypersensitivity to certain foods and chemicals, such as artificial colors and flavoring.

Just ask the parents of a child who has recovered from autism to describe their experience for you, or, better yet, ask a recovered child. You will gain a powerful insight: Sometimes when a health disorder is widely accepted as an "incurable genetic disease," it means only that medical doctors do not understand what is going on. Allopathic medicine has yet to concern itself with the profound yet subtle importance of toxicity and nutrient deficiency in human health and disease, despite our current knowledge that these factors influence the very expression of our genes.

The pharmacological status quo of health care is fighting to maintain its position as the true center of the health care universe, using its vast economic and political resources to discredit nonmedical strategies for health recovery, regardless of how well they may work.

The pharmaceutical/industrial complex, known variously as Big Pharma and the prescription drug cartel, was dubbed by Robert Mendelsohn, M.D., as the Church of Modern Medicine. "Once you understand Modern Medicine as a religion, you can fight it and defend yourself much more effectively than when you think you're fighting an art or a science…. Modern Medicine relies on faith to survive. All religions do. So heavily does the Church of Modern Medicine rely on faith that if everyone somehow simply forgot to believe in it for just one day, the whole system would collapse," wrote Mendelsohn in his book *Confessions of a Medical Heretic.*

Approximately 106,000 people die from properly prescribed medications in hospitals each year, reported the *Journal of the American Medical Association* in April 1998, and another 98,000 people die each year from medical errors, according the Institute of Medicine in its November 1999 report, *To Err is Human: Building a Safer Health System.*

To tackle this enormous problem, seven major drug companies and our own Food and Drug Administration (FDA) have recently pooled their resources to form a nonprofit organization called the International Serious Adverse Event Consortium (ISAEC). Could it be, though, that what we really need is an entirely different organization, one that focuses on helping all the people in our society become healthier without drugs? How about a nonprofit whose purpose is to celebrate our miraculous innate powers of healing and whose activities spread awareness of the many natural, nontoxic strategies that are known to enhance health on the cellular level? Perhaps we could call it the Innately Healthy Seriously Drug-Free Consortium.

But back to the ISAEC; I have not confirmed this, but presumably the goal of the organization is to reduce the sheer volume of death and disability caused annually by prescription drugs. If so, this is a very worthy goal, because the extent of the prescription drug problem is truly staggering. I wish these eminent scientists would realize that there is a simple solution to the problem, though I doubt if they will, and here's why: An adverse drug reaction is analogous to getting pregnant. The only surefire way to prevent pregnancy is complete abstinence. In the case of drugs, the only surefire way to avoid suffering the drug reaction is to abstain entirely from taking the drug in the first place. The possibility that ISAEC leaders will debate the merits of drug avoidance and explore natural healing strategies to forgo using drugs with their inherent risks of death and disability is about as remote as the moon itself.

And so it goes. Mother Nature's karma will inevitably run over the dogma of modern allopathic medicine, it is only a matter of time. In the meanwhile, I guess we will just have to get busy updating the textbooks, encourage the old leaders to take an early retirement, and never miss an opportunity to avoid prescription medication whenever possible.

Washing Our Hands of Swine Flu Hysteria

The undeserving maintain power by promoting hysteria.
Frank Herbert

For some reason we citizens of this great country are treated like mushrooms by our public health leaders. You know, kept in the dark and fed manure—in this case, pig manure. I am, of course, referring to the great swine flu pandemic debacle and the federal government's frantic promotion of the experimental H1N1 vaccine.

In 2009 our federal government and governments all around the world together declared that humankind was facing one of the biggest health threats in recorded history. At that time, the most distinctive thing about the H1N1 swine flu virus was its dreary and lackluster quality, and its propensity to be tame and below average as influenza viruses go. But on June 11, 2009, the World Health Organization (WHO) punched the big red hyperpanic button for the swine flu, triggering a global chain reaction of emergency medical preparations.

A Phase 6 Global Pandemic Alert, until that moment, stood as the highest possible red-flag warning, reserved only for the most massively monstrous and hideously harmful epidemic. So WHO moved the goal-post? At some point earlier in 2009, the term "global pandemic" was redefined by the WHO on its Web site, resulting in a dramatic, instant upgrade for the piggy virus from puny pathogen to perilous pandemic.

The WHO's prior definition of pandemic had always stated that influenza pandemics cause "enormous numbers of deaths and illness," but for reasons best known to the WHO leadership, the phrase describing death and illness was deleted from its Web site in the spring of 2009. The actions of the WHO and its member governments ratcheted up fear about the new flu to just south of extreme panic.

Panic did indeed break out in a few countries, such as India, but with so many other fundamental problems to deal with, such as trying to get food to feed the family, much of world's population reacted with apathy to the new flu fear.

This may explain why the WHO felt compelled to fire off hysteria-laden press releases every few days. A typical update warned that the H1N1 flu was spreading at an "unbelievable speed," and horror of horrors, a few turkeys in Chile were suffering with the virus. In case anyone failed to realize just how serious things were getting, the WHO repeatedly reminded governments they "must prepare for the worst."

"Whatever hysteria exists is inflamed by mystery, suspicion and secrecy. Hard and exact facts will cool it," wrote Elia Kazan, words befitting all the swine flu fabrications.

Just how bad did the swine flu get here in the United States? From CBS News, hardly a bastion of criticism for mainstream medicine, came this assessment: "If you have been diagnosed 'probable' or 'presumed' 2009 H1N1 or 'swine flu' in recent months, you may be surprised to know this: odds are you didn't have the H1N1 flu. In fact, you probably didn't have flu at all."

Wait a minute, wasn't the government shrieking that "virtually all" cases of flu were swine flu? Who was tracking the terrible pandemic flu? Not the government, it turns out.

The Centers for Disease Control (CDC) advised all fifty states in late July 2009 to stop counting individual cases of H1N1 flu, and to stop all testing for H1N1 flu, period. The official reason: Why waste resources on confirming cases of swine flu when we already know we are in the midst of a raging pandemic?

Wait a minute. Was it possible our health leaders had substantial evidence that CBS News did not know about, new data verifying that swine flu was sweeping the nation? In a word, no. CBS News requested specific information from the CDC about the stop order but received no response. CBS next filed a Freedom of Information Act request with the Department of Health and Human Services (HHS) but still heard nothing for over two months.

In the meantime, CBS contacted all fifty states and asked for their cumulative flu-tracking statistics prior to the July directive from the government to stop counting influenza cases. The details that emerged from the states' confirmed counts sharply contradicted the bellowing and arm waving coming from our health authorities. Based on actual testing, only a teensy-weensy number of swine flu cases were in evidence.

According to CBS, "The vast majority of cases were negative for H1N1 as well as seasonal flu, despite the fact that many states were specifically testing patients deemed to be most likely to have H1N1 flu, based on symptoms and risk factors."

Not only did these people not have the swine flu, the vast majority of those tested were not suffering from influenza virus of any kind—they just had flu-like symptoms. In California the tests showed 86 percent of tested samples were not influenza at all, and only 2 percent were H1N1. Georgia's testing also indicated that only 2 percent of the samples were positive for H1N1 flu. In Alaska, 93 percent of the samples were not influenza of any kind, with only 1 percent being H1N1. Florida reported the highest percentage, with 17 percent of samples confirmed as swine flu.

Despite the fact that swine flu cases were rather difficult to find anywhere in the country, this alarming headline was typical during the height of the hysteria: "H1N1 Flu Infects 250 Georgetown Students." But when CBS investigated the facts, it turned out that the number 250 was merely the number of students complaining of flu-like symptoms who had either visited the student health center, called the health center's H1N1 hotline, or visited the hospital's emergency room. Not a single test to confirm influenza was done on any of the students. A more accurate headline would have read, 250 Georgetown Students Complain of Flu-Like Illness, National Trends Indicate Few Cases are Likely Swine Flu, Zero Cases of Influenza of Any Kind Confirmed at Georgetown.

Hundreds of presumptive swine flu headlines in the summer months of 2009 made it sound as if swine flu were rampaging across the nation like a galloping herd of death-dealing wild boars. Predictably, the result of this tide of blatant public health disinformation being unleashed upon our citizenry was a stampede of fearful people rushing to visit emergency medical facilities.

Hospitals and clinics all over the country were swamped with folks worried sick they were suffering the dreaded H1N1 flu. Based on rapid, in-office tests for the flu, many of these people might actually have had influenza of some type, but was it swine flu? Based on the tests being used, we will never know.

"The rapid tests do not tell if a patient has the swine flu. They say only if flu is present, or in some cases whether it is type A or type B influenza. The swine flu is type A, but so are many seasonal flu strains," said the New York Times.

CDC's order to stop detailed tracking of flu cases surprised and per-plexed many seasoned public health experts, such as Dr. Bela Matyas, California's Acting Chief of Emergency Preparedness and Response. "With CDC's fallback position, there are so many uncertainties with who's being counted, it's hard to know how much we're seeing is due to H1N1 flu rather than a mix of influenza diseases generally," Matyas told CBS.

If H1N1 influenza truly was affecting young people and pregnant mothers differently than seasonal flu, complete with the unusually high mortality rates being claimed by government sources, wouldn't precise tracking be vital in order to create intelligent responses based on the best available scientific data? Not only did we lack an accurate count of how many piggies were in the barn in the first place, it seems the fed-eral government was trying to close the proverbial barn door after all the sneaky swine had escaped.

"In this situation, where the virus has been circulating in the popu-lation for some time and the vaccines are just beginning to be available, it is shortsighted to imagine that mass immunization is going to make much difference to the outbreak," according to Philip Alcabes, infec-tious disease specialist at CUNY Hunter College. "It's shocking that in 2009, knowing what we know, our public health establishment still deals with the flu as if it were 1957," Alcabes told ABC News.

New Zealand and Australia, countries in the Southern Hemisphere whose flu season occurs six months ahead of ours, typically foreshadow the U.S. flu-season experience. Once the flu season ended in those countries in the year of the so-called pandemic, we knew that the death rate was lower than usual for a flu season, all of this prior to the avail-ability of any H1N1 vaccine whatsoever.

Nevertheless, swine flu stories were relentlessly recycled, rehashed, and repeated over the airwaves. Terribly deadly flu! Not enough vaccine! This strategy of persistent fear mongering about the flu is taken straight from the pages of the CDC's playbook of reliable methods to create demand for the flu shot, spelled out in an official CDC document called (I am not making this up), "The Seven-Step Recipe for Generating Interest in, and Demand for, Flu (or any other) Vaccination."

In May 2009 HHS director Robin Robinson promised the Washington Post that the government's plans for mass vaccination would be scaled back if the H1N1 pandemic "fizzles out." But because the government deliberately eliminated even the slightest shred of scientific tracking, it was impossible to tell whether the pandemic was sizzling, fizzling, or just lightly drizzling, even as an emergency plan for mass vaccination of the entire populous was cranked up to full throttle.

Leaders in the Obama administration played their role with gusto, warning that 90,000 Americans would likely die in the fall of 2009 because of swine flu infections, while millions would be terribly sick and 300,000 would wind up in the intensive care ward.

The U.S. government wasted no time writing checks totaling more than $1.6 billion to a handful of vaccine makers for 229 million flu shots, scribbling faster than you can say "mercury toxicity." Officials were also quick to begin distributing billions of dollars of stockpiled antiviral drugs as the best defense against the new flu.

Ah yes, the antivirals. What was known at the time about the ability of the antivirals to fight viruses? First, viruses frequently become resistant to these drugs quite rapidly, thereby providing no benefit at all. Second, in those cases when the antiviral actually "works," it simply means that flu symptoms might begin easing off sooner—by less than a day.

And what of the safety of antivirals? The number of known adverse reactions to Tamiflu, in particular, was already significant. In Japan the drug was banned for teenagers because of an increased risk of suicidal behavior. Tamiflu's own safety information stated: "People with the flu, particularly children and adolescents, may be at an increased risk of self-injury and confusion shortly after taking Tamiflu and should be closely monitored."

Critics of the government's swine flu fanaticism said it was swine flu déjà vu, a repeat of the 1976 swine flu-vaccine disaster. In that year 40 million people were injected with a fast-tracked, untested vaccine, resulting in 25 deaths and 500 cases of paralysis from Guillain-Barre syndrome, all for one "probable" (unconfirmed) case of swine flu. Thousands of legal claims were filed seeking compensation for vaccine-induced injuries, and taxpayers coughed up more than $1.3 billion in awards for death and damages caused by the vaccine that year.

Fast-forward to 2009: CDC officials were cheerfully chirping that the new fast-tracked, untested pandemic vaccines would surely be "just as safe as seasonal flu vaccines," which makes it sound as if the seasonal flu shot has actually been studied and its safety established for pregnant women and young children, the two groups placed by the government at the head of the line for the H1N1 flu shot. Unfortunately, seasonal flu vaccines have never been tested for safety for these populations.

"There is no study of the vaccines on pregnant women—no randomized clinical trials," according to researcher Tom Jefferson of the independently funded, highly regarded Cochrane Institute. And according to the printed insert for one brand of seasonal influenza vaccine, "Safety and effectiveness of Flulaval have not been established in pregnant women, nursing mothers, and children."

Children with asthma who received another seasonal vaccine, Flu-Mist (the up-your-nose flu vaccine), experienced a threefold increased risk of hospitalization, according to a study presented at the 2009 American Thoracic Society International Conference. Would other surprises be in store for us once the safety studies of the H1N1 vaccine were finally—if ever—done?

Even as pregnant women were being vaccinated with the now-available, still-untested H1N1 vaccine, one clinical trial was begun, sponsored by the National Institute of Allergy and Infectious Disease (NIAID). Recruitment was under way to find pregnant women for a randomized trial—randomized but not placebo controlled. What? Believe it or not, standard procedure in vaccine safety trials is scientifically substandard, pure and simple. Why? Because the very first rule of authentic scientific investigation gets thrown out the window at the outset of every single vaccine safety trial: Use of an actual placebo with a control group is *never* part of the trials. Ever. In classic premeditated, fixed-outcome pseudo-science, the NIAID study was set up to simply compare the safety of one flu shot to another flu shot. Each vaccine contains a bewildering array of toxic chemicals, foreign proteins, and heavy metals. Any adverse reactions common to both vaccines gets reported as "perfectly safe by comparison."

This is known as cigarette science, the best science money can buy, made to order for hiding the inherent dangers of using a product as intended. It is the same as comparing one group of pregnant smokers with another group of pregnant smokers, while meticulously documenting zero difference in health between the two groups. The point of the whole exercise is to be able to blast the headlines around the world at the conclusion of the study, "Smoking cigarettes found perfectly safe for pregnant women and their babies." In this case we can simply replace "smoking cigarettes" with "flu shots."

Dr. Marie Paul Kieny, director of vaccine research at the WHO, explained what was known and not known about the safety of the untested pandemic flu shots in 2009 this way: "It's not to say they would not be safe, they may be very safe but there is no data for the time being to demonstrate safety." Translated into ordinary English, this means no one knows diddly-squat about the effects of the shot. Ready! Fire! Aim!

The following draft statement from the federal government's Vaccine Advisory Committee was a bald-faced admission that we were embarking on a massive, risky, medical experiment involving millions of human guinea pigs in the United States: "The need to actively monitor vaccine recipients for vaccine adverse events is critical given that the vaccine candidates will all contain a new antigen and may be combined with adjuvants that are not part of licensed vaccines in the U.S."

Here's one thing we learned about the effects of the European formulation of the shot after the fact: "The vaccine is now suspected to be linked to an increase in the number of cases of narcolepsy affecting children and young people in Finland, Sweden and Iceland. In Finland, 54 children have been diagnosed with narcolepsy," said the Chief Medical Officer of Finland's Public Health Service, Dr. Terhi Kilpi. Had she known ahead of time of the risks, no recommendation for five- to twenty-year-olds to receive the shot would have been made, she said.

And how well did the U.S. government "actively monitor vaccine recipients for vaccine adverse events" as promised? Well, according to Dr. Marie McCormick of the CDC, there were zero vaccine-related adverse events in pregnant women caused by the vaccine. But her claim is rather amazing considering that an independent assessment of the government's own Vaccine Adverse Event Reporting System (VAERS) database carried out by the National Coalition of Organized Women found a 700 percent increase over nonpandemic years in stillbirths for pregnant women who were given the H1N1 vaccine. Such a radical discrepancy suggests that the CDC is more interested in promoting flu shots than examining unintended tragic health consequences caused by the shots.

And we simply cannot ignore the enormous gap in the logic—approximately the width of the Grand Canyon—that was used to justify vaccinating as many people as possible as soon as possible. Since the virus itself was proving to be more harmless than the average seasonal flu bug, all the excitement about the virus was based on fear. It was the fear that H1N1 might mutate and become something entirely different, a dangerous virus. Such a mutation was a definite possibility, but the H1N1 vaccine concoction was produced using the premutation, feeble virus, not the fearfully dreaded something-else-that-might-evolve virus. Therefore, if the dreaded mutation did take place and H1N1 did manage to change itself into a formidable virus, the fast-tracked premutation inoculation would be useless in stimulating an effective immune response.

Not so, said vaccine defenders, who are of the opinion that injecting an influenza strain "close" to mutated versions offers "some protection." Understandably, this hypothesis is very popular with flu-shot promoters, but no scientific support for this argument has been produced. Among our health leaders it is a matter of consensus that the hypothetical "some protection" factor is a firmly established scientific principle. Translated, consensus means: Screw the science. We are really important and powerful people and we make up the rules as we see fit. All who disagree that flu shots are safe and effective are idiots.

Those same health leaders experienced grave disappointment in the small number of people who could be frightened into getting stuck with the H1N1 shot. It seems the majority of the American public can tell when public health measures are utterly lacking in scientific integrity and common sense. Even as the H1N1 story unraveled and the fabricated danger of swine flu toppled under its own weight, our health leaders kept shoveling on more, uh, swine excreta.

"Unfortunately we are seeing more illness, more hospitalizations, and more deaths," said Anne Schuchat, M.D., director of the CDC's National Center for Immunization and Respiratory Diseases. Schuchat blamed swine flu for "virtually all" the flu cases in 2009. We now know that this declaration was made in the utter absence of any verifiable scientific data. In fact, the evidence that we do have suggests that the exact opposite was true. Apparently, "mathematical modeling" is now a sufficient basis for generating pandemic hysteria.

It has become apparent that all it takes to fuel the mighty flu-vaccine juggernaut is hot air. Just days before Halloween 2009, in the grand tradition of tricking and treating, the CDC released newly made-up numbers that proved things were way worse than reported in earlier made-up numbers: "By the end of July, up to 5.7 million Americans—140 times the reported number—had H1N1 swine flu," according to

WebMd. Yup, and I can personally guarantee that these numbers were carefully studied by Daffy Duck and verified by Porky Pig.

Lost in all the flu hysteria—swine and seasonal—is truly important news: positive, noninvasive, nontoxic, health-building steps; steps that can actually help us avoid all infections, influenza or not, are well within the reach of even the most modest household budget. Namely, we need to exercise some common sense and stop worrying about getting sick. Get outdoors and exercise, get plenty of rest, eat a healthy and diverse diet of wholesome, living foods free of chemical contaminants, drink plenty of pure water, and supplement with high-quality vitamins A, C, D, and E as well as magnesium.

Independent research reproduced the world over tells us that these measures are safe and remarkably effective. Is it too much to hope that official pronouncements will someday inform the public about how to build up health to help us face any flu, old or new? Or is it better for health authorities to run around in circles screaming that the sky is falling—or rather the sky might theoretically begin falling soon if a few storm clouds somehow appeared out of a clear blue sky and become a dangerous, life-threatening storm?

The public needs to be reassured that the relatively small number of deaths associated with the H1N1 virus in the United States involved individuals with underlying health challenges. Our knowledge of which populations are at risk of death following influenza infection is scarcely a mystery: Influenza virus may be dangerous for persons with weak or compromised immune systems, but, historically, to the average well-nourished healthy person, influenza poses little mortal risk.

The same cannot be said, however, of certain vaccine ingredients, such as mercury, aluminum phosphate, and formaldehyde, each one harmful to human health 100 percent of the time, even in trace amounts.

Despite the farcical, fizzled, farmyard flu pandemic, all around the world there is talk of forcing health-care workers—without exception—to get stuck with the seasonal flu and H1N1 shots or lose their jobs. Ordinary citizens, according to public health leaders, should be pressured to get the flu shot under the threat of lost civil liberties. Even so, more and more people are just saying no. Recent polls of nurses and doctors indicate many will continue refusing the shot, and the public continues stubbornly resisting the siren call of the flu-shot enthusiasts.

In place of crying "wolf!" our health leaders this time cried "swine!" The betrayal of public trust in this flu fable comes with a huge price tag, as discovered by the boy in the Aesop's fable. Our health leaders may find even greater public apathy next time they squeal, "Hey everybody listen to us! Please! We really mean it this time!"

As alarming as it is to witness gross incompetence and blatant dishonesty from those charged with protection of the public's health, there are some valuable lessons we can we take away from the swine flu non-pandemic. Number one is to recognize that "the flu" is flu-like illness the vast majority of the time and usually not an influenza virus at all.

Tom Jefferson, M.D., of the Cochrane Institute has offered some sensible suggestions. "We need a more comprehensive and perhaps more effective strategy in controlling acute respiratory infections, relying on several preventive interventions that take into account the multi-agent nature of infectious respiratory disease and its context" such as personal hygiene, adequate food, pure water and sanitary living conditions.

I suggest that several billion dollars and a lot of trouble could be saved in the next flu-for-all using a more "calculated" response. The only signs of danger amidst all the pandemic pandemonium arose from mathematical modeling, so the next time they throw a pandemic, the only people we really need to inoculate are the government mathematicians and vaccine policy makers.

For the rest of us, it is time to wash our hands of flu hysteria. Rest assured that hysteria-provoking mathematical models are neither highly infectious nor deadly—unless we get scared and actually start believing them. Oh, and one more thing, avoid pro-flu shot experts and government statisticians like the plague. But if you mistakenly come in contact with one, be sure to wash your hands with soap.

Two Causes: Too Much, Too Little

Happiness is a way station between too little and too much.

Channing Pollock

There are so many diseases to choose from these days that no one seems to know exactly how many diseases there are. One medical expert I asked told me there are at least 10,000 different health disorders that have their own name. By remarkable coincidence, many of these diseases were discovered and described just before a new prescription medication was approved and marketed to treat the newly named disorder.

But just like everything else in life, the answer to the question of how many diseases there are depends upon whom you ask. For example, if you asked the cells in your body how many there are, without any hesitation they would answer, "There are only two diseases." Believe it or not, your cells operate under the assumption there are only two diseases: One is called Too Much, and the other is called Too Little.

I know this may sound rather simple-minded, foolish and hopelessly naïve, but everyone is entitled to their opinion, including the 70 trillion or so life units that comprise the human body. How dare those tiny little human cells go around claiming to know more about health than medical professionals, who, after all, have attended real medical schools, have real diplomas hanging on their walls, and are licensed to prescribe really dangerous drugs? But there's no stopping those miraculous, microscopic mavericks. Those little pipsqueaks would have us believe that the body's innate wisdom and ability to organize health far surpasses that of doctors and drug companies. Such arrogance.

One thing on which the pharmaceutical industry and our cells can agree is that all processes in the body are based on chemistry. Cells are chemical factories that are organized by the central nervous system to maintain the delicate balance of body chemistry inside the body from one nanosecond to the next. The pharmaceutical industry makes a wide variety of patented chemical formulations called drugs, and these are used to intentionally alter some aspect of the body's innate chemistry.

And yet every single thing we do changes the body's chemistry. Our rate of breathing, exercising, resting, eating food, drinking beverages, even the thoughts we think affect body chemistry. When body chemistry is balanced, human activities have the best chance of being at peak function. This includes cellular growth and repair, the healing of tissues and organs, coordination, endurance, creativity, and even success in relationships.

At any given moment each cell inside the human body is either (a) growing and repairing itself or (b) defending and guarding itself. No cell is capable of both growing and guarding itself simultaneously. However, within the human body, among the trillions of cells, some cells may be in health-building mode while other cells are on defensive alert, depleting rather than producing resources.

Which brings us to the concept of too much—of anything: food, carbon dioxide, oxygen, toxins, even excess nerve signaling from irritated nerves. Getting too much of any of these tends to create interference with normal, healthy cell function. Consider, for example, someone who drinks too much alcohol. Coordination, thinking, speaking, and judgment (not to mention driving) all become impaired when the body's cells have to cope with too much alcohol sloshing around, until the kidneys are able to filter and eliminate the alcohol from the blood and the whole body system.

Alcohol and other chemical toxins are often described as "harmless" in small amounts, even though the same substance may be deadly in a slightly greater quantity. The cells' side of the story tells us that this thinking is not exactly correct. Certain substances are so toxic that even the smallest exposure will cause some cells to switch to defensive mode, thereby ending their growth and repair activities. Depending on the toxin and the dose, a certain number of cells will even die.

A toxin or chemical by tradition is called "safe" when the rate of cell disruption and cell death caused by the substance is at or below an "acceptable" level of damage. For example, heavy alcohol consumption most definitely kills a certain number of brain cells but does not necessarily kill the person, unless a certain threshold of toxicity is reached. For other substances, such as formaldehyde, there is no safe level of ingestion or exposure for humans at all, according to the Environmental Protection Agency. That is because the level of cell disruption and cell death is too high. (Isn't it interesting that formaldehyde is an ingredient in many vaccines, all of which are said to be "safe" and are repeatedly injected into tiny humans.)

Too Little is the flip side of the health coin, according to our cells. This means there is a lack of vital nutrients necessary for healthy cellular activities such as respiration, ingestion, excretion and chemical manufacture. If there is a shortage of a vital nutrient, first there will be disorder and dysfunction in the cells. Next, there will be disorder in the tissues comprising those cells. These conditions lead to dysfunction of the organ made up of the troubled tissue and finally develop into disease processes in the whole body. By contrast, when the proper nutrients are available to cells in the proper quantities at the proper time, the miracle of good health simply "happens" in the body.

Biologists estimate that within 1 square inch of skin there are 1,300 nerve cells, 4 yards of nerve fibers, 100 sweat glands, and 3 yards of blood vessels. During the time it takes you to read this paragraph, about 50 million cells in your body will have died and been replaced. For most people, the entire body is renewed on the cellular level every couple of years. If an individual's replacement cells are healthy, it bodes well for his or her overall health.

The body possesses an amazing innate intelligence that automatically controls and regulates temperature, blood pressure, breathing, heart rate, and blood chemistry at every moment, night and day, awake and asleep. A balance of body chemistry, regulated by the body's innate wisdom and controlled by the central nervous system, delivers just the right quantity and quality of the body's own chemicals in exactly the right place at precisely the right moment. Think of the body as nature's perfect pharmacy.

The two-disease theory is alive and well among cells; it always has been and always will be. It is also popular among a growing number of health professionals who find that focusing on building up health at the cellular level allows people to regain their health naturally without risk of unintended consequences or adverse drug reactions.

Simplicity is defined in the world of engineering as the degree to which a system or component has a design and implementation that is straightforward and easy to understand.

As long as we are able to hold onto our health freedom, we are each free to decide whether our cells' story of too much and too little is simple-minded foolishness—or rather the shimmering magnificence of nature's elegant simplicity. When it comes to health and healing, the explanation with the greatest simplicity seems to reveal the greatest wisdom of all.

Innate Healing and Nutritional Intervention

Man is a food-dependent creature. If you don't feed him, he will die.
If you feed him improperly, part of him will die.

Emanuel Cheraskin, M.D.

Whether the American public knows it or not, much of the medical advice we receive comes from doctors with a peculiar specialty: spinning. Spin doctors have emerged as the most powerful of doctors in the allopathic medical world—master manipulators of facts, fabricators of fear, and pushers of pills through pharmaceutical advertising. The constant barrage of drug advertising in our country feeds the public a daily diet of misinformation/disinformation claiming that we are all suffering diseases caused by bad luck and faulty genes and that the real underlying problem is a deficiency of prescription medication.

But no amount of pharmaceutical advertising can alter the principle that humans are born innately capable of creating excellent health, given the proper resources. If our cells are not quite up to optimal health, our body is striving to make it so. To the extent that we are able to assist our innate healing, we create our own wellness.

Sadly, the term wellness has become nearly cliché, its meaning twisted and distorted to fit a variety of health and early detection strategies of questionable value, but it remains the best term we have for now.

A wellness approach to living is one that seeks to supply the body with an abundance of the nutrients it needs, in a healthy, nurturing environment, together with an active lifestyle that helps the body thrive. Wellness is not simply the absence of disease, but a state of constantly engaging in habits and activities to achieve well-being. This goes far beyond survival, to "thrival." Thrival is described as a state of positive emotional and spiritual life, plenty of outdoor activities and exercise, avoiding toxic inputs, and surrounding oneself with love and gratitude. The question asked by wellness is this: What can I do every day to help my cells, tissues, organs—my whole body and mind—move in the direction of optimal health?

At the other extreme of the health care spectrum is allopathy, the treatment of disease through the use of drugs to suppress symptoms. The question asked by allopathic disease management is this: Which drug, or combination of drugs, best alleviates the symptom or mitigates the negative clinical finding (such as high blood pressure) with the least amount of unwanted adverse effects? The hidden question inherent in this approach is this: What other drugs do I need to take to suppress the unwanted symptoms caused by the medications I'm already taking?

A wellness approach necessarily spends an inordinate amount of time considering, planning, and preparing food. The nutritional quality of our food supply has steadily deteriorated over the last several decades as agriculture has become industrialized and our food has become intensely processed, refined, and denatured. Food today is long on shelf life and chemical additives, but short on nutritional value. It is likely no mere coincidence that epidemics of chronic health disorders have steadily increased just as food quality has decreased. It is no longer a viable option to rely on food alone to supply us with the nutrients we need—unless we live on organic farms and raise our own produce and livestock.

"We consume the elements of our own destruction, with our excessive intake of sugar and unsaturated fats, loss of bulk or fiber, elimination of vitamins and minerals, and pollution of food with chemicals never demonstrated to be safe," according to nutrition pioneer Abram Hoffer, M.D., "But when the sick population includes sufferers from senility, cardiovascular conditions, arthritis, schizophrenia, learning and behavioral disorders, cancer of the colon, peptic ulcer and many other individual problems, society seems not to add them together as one major problem."

The realization that chronic nutritional deficiencies constitute the basic underlying problem in chronic illness is slowly penetrating the mindset of the allopathic medical community, along with the logical conclusion that nutritional intervention can frequently be used in place of medical intervention to help patients heal themselves. A recent indicator of this trend was in evidence at the U.S. Food and Drug Administration, when the agency acknowledged that many prescription drugs cause hypomagnesemia (a deficiency of magnesium), a serious problem that must be remedied immediately with supplementation.

Unfortunately, it is still the case that docs who stray too far from their pharmaceutical prescription pads and prescribe instead a pathway of wellness frequently find themselves in trouble with their professional associations and medical boards for unprofessional conduct.

The real changes in health care are coming from health care consumers. I predict that before long we will reach the tipping point. That will happen when a sufficient number of people understand that a combination of eating nutritious foods, staying active, and using nutritional supplements will allow them to avoid many conditions currently treated with drug intervention. When those millions of people seize the day and reclaim their own innate healing, drug companies will be in big trouble. But as long as the mainstream media looks to Big Pharma sources for health-related news, stories about vitamins and their role in helping people heal will likely remain starkly inaccurate.

Of course, the vitamin story would be far different if vitamins could be patented. Pharmaceutical companies would be making and marketing those little pills like there was no tomorrow if they held patents on vital nutrients. I can guarantee that as you read this, pharmaceutical researchers are busy in drug laboratories tweaking natural vitamin molecules with the goal of creating patented supplements. In the meantime, the industry strategy seems to consist of mounting repeated attacks on the safety and effectiveness of vitamins.

A typical hit piece against vitamins appeared in the *Journal of the American Medical Association* (JAMA) in January 2007. This study concluded that taking certain individual antioxidants not only fails to help you live longer, it may even shorten your life.

The average medical doctor, trained to believe that drugs and nutrients are best studied in an identical fashion, fails to recognize the fundamental error in such studies. A randomized clinical trial design used to evaluate vitamins would typically give one group of people a single antioxidant supplement and the other group a placebo.

But this approach to testing individual nutrients is patently absurd. The body needs the whole team of nutrients the same way a coach needs the whole football team to win the game. Biochemical pathways that enable the absorption and utilization of one nutrient are derived from other specific nutrients, which require other nutrients, and so on and on in complex biochemical cycles and feedback loops.

Would the quarterback ever be sent onto the field to face the entire opposing team all by himself? Of course not. Winning the health game depends on having the entire team of vital nutrients present at all times, each member contributing maximum levels of performance. The human body requires a balanced supply of each and every nutrient, and only then can all systems function properly to produce energy and build healthy cells. It is important to note that the stresses we all encounter in daily life on occasion deplete certain nutrients, which increases the demand for those nutrients.

The recent article published in JAMA casting doubt on the value of nutritional supplements proves one thing only: The results of research can only be as good as the questions being asked in the study.

Suppose researchers had asked a better question, such as this: Do people who consume antioxidants as part of a healthy lifestyle that includes eating a balanced diet of fresh, uncontaminated food and regular exercise enjoy a higher quality of life and greater longevity with a reduced need for medical intervention? I'm guessing that the conclusions to a study based on this question would be significantly different.

After all, the importance of good nutrition for good health is not exactly breaking news. More than 2,000 years ago Hippocrates advised, "Let thy food be thy medicine, and thy medicine be thy food."

But it wasn't until 1757 that Scottish physician James Lind became the first person to demonstrate a direct link between a major illness and lack of a specific nutrient. Using one of the first controlled medical experiments in history, Lind showed that sailors supplied with citrus fruits and sauerkraut were able to avoid the telltale signs of scurvy. The symptoms include bleeding gums, rough skin, muscle weakness, poor wound healing, anemia, and death.

British navy Captain James Cook soon became the first ship commander to take Lind's advice and require his sailors to eat quantities of citrus fruits and pickled vegetables during long voyages to prevent scurvy. This practice was successful and became policy throughout the British navy, earning British sailors the nickname "limeys" (which is perhaps preferable to "lemonys" or "fruitys").

We now recognize scurvy as vitamin C deficiency disorder. Other so-called incurable diseases were later found to result from underlying deficiencies of other specific nutrients. In this manner vitamins were discovered one by one, and we wiped out deficiency diseases such as beriberi, pellagra and rickets; all gone except for those individuals who do not receive adequate nutrition.

The practice of prescribing very high doses of vitamins to treat so-called incurable cases of various diseases is the realm of orthomolecular medicine. The Orthomolecular Society describes orthomolecular medicine as the practice of preventing and treating disease by giving the body optimal amounts of substances that are natural to the body. Two-time Nobel Prize winner Linus Pauling, Ph.D., coined the term "orthomolecular" in 1968, meaning "right molecule."

The orthomolecular view is neatly summed up in a question asked by Emanuel Cheraskin, M.D., "Why is it so many of us are 40 going on 70, and so few 70 going on 40?" He believes the answer to that question is our neglect of the importance of nutrition, which he calls an educational deficiency.

The practice of orthomolecular medicine has an amazing track record of safety and effectiveness. Its list of disciples includes several Nobel Prize laureates. Tragically, orthomolecular medicine is dismissed by members of the allopathic medical community and periodically attacked. Mysteriously, orthomolecular medicine is also excluded from Medline, our nation's taxpayer-funded public medical literature index.

Medline is the online index of the U.S. National Library of Medicine, an arm of the National Institutes of Health (NIH). "The subject scope of Medline is biomedicine and health, broadly defined to encompass those areas of the life sciences, behavioral sciences, chemical sciences, and bioengineering needed by health professionals and others engaged in basic research and clinical care, public health, health policy development, or related educational activities," according to the NIH's Web site.

Medline includes more than 5,000 journals in the index, so why exclude the *Journal of Orthomolecular Medicine*, a peer-reviewed journal in publication for more than 40 years? "The National Library of Medicine refuses to index the *Journal of Orthomolecular Medicine*, though it is peer-reviewed and seems to meet their criteria," reported *Psychology Today* in November 2006.

Is it possible that the folks at the National Library of Medicine are attempting to censor high-quality research that describes successful treatment of such diverse health disorders as autism, schizophrenia, multiple sclerosis, Huntington's disease, bipolar disorder, cancer, and shingles using orthomolecular principles and protocols?

In tiny, tiny amounts, vitamins prevent deadly diseases such as scurvy and pellagra, yet at 1,000 times the effective dosage and even higher, most vitamins are still nontoxic. Even so, medical doctors are strongly advised to adhere to the "official" minimum nutrient levels; levels that are calculated to be just sufficient to prevent the symptoms of deficiency disease. Would these same doctors consider for even a moment driving around in their imported luxury cars while maintaining the oil level just slightly above the threshold of severe engine damage? I don't think so.

Luckily, clinicians all over the world are focusing on nutritional intervention and successfully helping people heal themselves from such disorders as mental illness, heart disease, autoimmune disease, and even cancer using the principle of abundantly supplying cells with specific cellular nutrients. These doctors recognize that most individuals with health challenges have specific and unique nutritional needs, far above the absolute minimum levels of officialdom.

I am told that the human species on this planet is collectively so sick with chronic disease that we belong on the endangered species list. Then why is it that anthropologists who study hunter/gatherer societies in the wild document a universal lack of heart disease, obesity, diabetes, stroke, and even tooth decay in such "backward" populations? Are we to believe that people living in the wild are born with a genetic makeup superior to those of us living in industrialized societies, or that their good health is due to exceptionally good luck?

Chronic disease is lifestyle induced, and it can be corrected only with lifestyle intervention. The development of chronic disease requires years of dedicated self-destructive behavior and poor habits. In many cases, individuals are unaware that over the course of their lifetimes they were creating their own health problems. That is why it is so vital that children learn at an early age that lifestyle choices profoundly affect future health.

The principle of wellness is the practice of honoring the daily miracle of innate healing, witnessing the laws of nature in action, and doing that which supports those laws. Just as the health of a rain forest depends on the health of the individual trees, so does the health of the body depend on the collective health of the individual cells.

There are three factors generally under our control that have a tremendous influence on our health. What kinds of thoughts occupy our minds? What things do we eat, drink, or otherwise put into our bodies? How well and how much do we keep our bodies in motion?

"The evidence is overwhelming that physical activity and diet can reduce the risk of developing numerous chronic diseases, including CAD [coronary artery disease], hypertension, diabetes, metabolic syndrome, and several forms of cancer, and in many cases in fact reverse existing disease," according to the *Journal of Applied Physiology* in January 2005. These disorders account for the vast majority of cases of preventable death each year in modern industrialized countries.

In an emergency, when the body is broken and failing, an allopathic medical response to suppress symptoms with drugs and/or surgery is entirely appropriate, but to continue with those interventions in the hopes of restoring the body to good health makes no sense. Here's the question: Suppose your house was damaged by fire. The day after the firemen arrived at your house with sirens blaring, smashed in the doors and windows, and drenched the whole house with water in order to successfully extinguish the fire, should you call them back to bring their axes and fire hoses and keep pouring water on the house and smashing things? No. At that point you need to eliminate the initial causes of the fire, as well as bring in carpenters, roofers, electricians, plumbers, painters, and others who can help build up the health of the house. Allopathic medicine can be excellent for putting out the fires in the body, but it provides little in the way of bodily repair and healing.

Innate healing is your birthright and organizes the health of your body from conception to your final breath. Healthy nutrition and healthy lifestyle choices allow the innate wisdom within our bodies to get back to work building up the health of the body as only Mother Nature can.

In the immortal words of Hippocrates, "If we could give every individual the right amount of nourishment and exercise, not too little and not too much, we would have found the safest way to health."

The Wait-and-See Earache Prescription

Everything comes if a man will only wait.
Benjamin Disraeli

Earaches bring more unhappy children to emergency rooms and pediatric offices each year than just about any other health disorder. Antibiotics remain the most popular medical treatment for earache, with doctors writing 15 million prescriptions for earache each year in the United States alone, according to the *Journal of the American Medical Association* (JAMA) September 2006.

Earache is the most common childhood ailment for which antibiotics are prescribed, even though most earaches are caused by viral, not bacterial infections, and 81 percent of infections heal nicely with no medication at all, according to the U.S. Department of Health and Human Services.

Due to the widespread overuse of antibiotics, drug-resistant germs have been reproducing as fast as frolicking bunnies, rapidly evolving to new heights of drug resistance. For more than a decade, health leaders have been sounding the alarm, trying to convince doctors to stop writing so many antibiotic prescriptions because of growing drug resistance, as well as the potentially serious damage to the health of people who take the drugs.

"The risks of antibiotics, including gastrointestinal symptoms, allergic reactions, and accelerated resistance to bacterial pathogens, must be weighed against their benefits for an illness that, for the most part, is self-limited," according to the authors of the JAMA study.

Antibiotics are potent weapons intended to annihilate select groups of offensive bacteria. Unfortunately, when antibiotics are taken, most of the hardworking, friendly bacteria in the body get slaughtered at the same time, wiping out the body's mighty microbe population that normally does important work inside, such as digesting food and making vitamin K.

The earache study published in JAMA was a test of a strategy called the "wait-and-see prescription" to help kids with earaches. This method has been around for a long time, but this was the first time it was tested in an emergency-room setting.

Half of the 283 children in the study diagnosed with acute otitis media (AOM) were sent home with a standard prescription, the other half with the wait-and-see prescription (WASP). The only difference between the two groups was that the parents in the WASP group were told to wait at least 48 hours before filling the antibiotic prescription.

An unbelievable two out of three children avoided antibiotics with the wait-and-see prescription. "The WASP approach substantially reduced unnecessary use of antibiotics in children with AOM seen in an emergency department and may be an alternative to routine use of antimicrobials for treatment of such children," was the understated conclusion of the study.

The WASP concept may well be one of the greatest advances in medical science since the discovery of the fundamental importance of hand washing. The immediate benefit will be in the fight against two very pressing medical problems, microbial drug resistance caused by widespread antibiotic misuse and abuse, and antibiotic-induced chronic gastrointestinal disease. But I can imagine other applications of wait and see throughout the medical profession. How about "wait-and-see surgery"?

The WASP study has been criticized because it is not a clinical randomized trial, which is considered the gold standard in medical science.

Researchers tend to believe that you might as well use the paper on which anecdotal case studies are written to line the floor of your birdcage. Out in the field, however, clinical practitioners place great value on case studies and observational evidence because of their usefulness in determining what works and what does not work to overcome a given health challenge.

Which brings up the phenomenon of parents bringing children with earache to the chiropractor's office. It is the number-one reason parents first bring their child to a chiropractor. How is it possible for chiropractic adjustments to help a child's ear heal? Recovery from an infection in the middle ear requires adequate liquid drainage through the eustachian tubes as well as lymphatic drainage through the lymph vessels. Nerve irritation in the cervical spine can cause abnormal tension in the neck muscles that inhibits normal opening and closing of the Eustachian tubes and restricts normal lymph drainage by compressing the lymph ducts.

"Chiropractic mobilizes drainage of the ear in children, and if they can continue to drain without a buildup of fluid and subsequent infection, they build up their own antibodies and recover more quickly," explains Joan Fallon, D.C.

Critics acknowledge that chiropractic care may be very popular with parents for their children who suffer earache but complain that the science verifying the chiropractic adjustment's ability to facilitate natural healing of the ears is inadequate. A number of case studies have been published that describe the neurological pathways involved and document the typical rapid recovery of earache under chiropractic care, but, alas, there have been no clinical randomized trials to date.

And that reminds me of the famous parachute study, published in the *British Medical Journal* in December 2003. According to the authors of this study, "parachutes are widely used to prevent death and major injury after gravitational challenge," yet the placebo-controlled randomized clinical trials have never been done. I'm thinking that at this point it may be difficult to find people willing to jump from an airplane wearing a placebo parachute. It looks and feels like the real thing when you put it on, but when you pull the cord nothing happens.

"The perception that parachutes are a successful intervention is based largely on anecdotal evidence....As with many interventions intended to prevent ill health, the effectiveness of parachutes has not been subjected to rigorous evaluation by using randomized controlled trials," wrote the authors.

Now I may be wrong, but it seems to me that people seeking good health are mostly interested in getting well as quickly as they can without having to worry about additional health risks. The wait-and-see prescription study does not suggest that parents and doctors should just ignore health problems and hope they go away, but it does provide additional evidence that when it comes to medical interventions, less is more.

Common sense suggests that if you need to jump out of a plane while still up in the air, you might want to strap on a real parachute without waiting for the double-blind studies. I agree with the authors of the JAMA study who concluded, "Individuals who insist that all interventions need to be validated by a randomized controlled trial need to come down to earth with a bump."

Coughing Up the Facts on Whooping Cough

> *The greatest enemy of the truth is very often not the lie—*
> *deliberate, contrived and dishonest, but the myth—*
> *persistent, persuasive and unrealistic.*
>
> John F. Kennedy

Every 3 to 5 years pertussis rolls into town and causes an outbreak of whooping cough. A whooping cough epidemic was declared in California on June 24, 2010. The most recent epidemic in California prior to that year was declared in 2005.

The Centers for Disease Control (CDC) tells us on its Web site that reported cases of whooping cough have been on the rise since the early 1980s, despite ever-increasing vaccination coverage. The number of babies less than 6 months old contracting pertussis continues to increase dramatically, even as the percentage of babies receiving the three-shot series at 2, 4, and 6 months old has steadily increased.

If more babies, kids, and adults than ever before are getting vaccinated against whooping cough, why are we seeing epidemics every few years? And why do fully vaccinated children and adults keep getting the whooping cough?

One explanation given is that vaccine effectiveness wanes over time. This is the rationale for additional shots and boosters periodically being added to the list of recommended vaccines, as well as recommendations to vaccinate and revaccinate older and older populations.

Another explanation is that we are seeing outbreaks of a different pertussis bacteria altogether, called parapertussis, with symptoms that are nearly identical to those of pertussis. Parapertussis is reportedly on the rise and is often mistaken for whooping cough, but no one knows to what extent. Lab tests are expensive, and most whooping cough cases are never laboratory confirmed; the diagnosis is usually based on symptoms alone.

The current state of affairs concerning recurring pertussis outbreaks raises some important questions. What exactly is whooping cough? What recommendations do public-health authorities make for protecting our babies? Are there other options? How do unvaccinated children fare during the periodic whooping cough outbreaks? Do unvaccinated children and adults cause the recurring outbreaks?

Whooping cough is a respiratory disease caused by toxins produced by the Bordetella pertussis bacteria. A strong immune response is typical, especially in the young, with production of large amounts of thick, sticky mucus that can block the breathing passageways of children and babies, making it difficult to breathe. The hallmark wrenching cough ends with the characteristic whooping sound as the child struggles to breathe, and this is often followed by vomiting. Babies typically show the classic whooping cough symptoms, whereas in older children and adults the symptoms often resemble only a bad cold.

Death from pertussis today is rare. Virtually all pertussis-related deaths occur in young people, with infants less than 6 months old accounting for 90 percent of deaths, according to the CDC. There were ten infant deaths in California attributed to whooping cough during the 2010 outbreak; all the babies were less than 3 months old.

In response to the cyclical outbreaks of whooping cough, the course of action promoted by state and federal public-health authorities is predictable: more shots. This time around, many public-health authorities once again blamed the epidemic on parents who opt out of vaccinating their kids, even though the percentage of children receiving the vaccine has steadily increased for decades.

"Pertussis, an acute, infectious cough illness, remains endemic in the United States despite routine childhood pertussis vaccination for more than half a century and high coverage levels in children for more than a decade." This statement from the CDC was made 10 years ago, so we are now talking about two decades of high rates of vaccination. Vaccine compliance for pertussis remains very high today, with at least 84 percent of children having completed the series of four shots by age three.

"The rise in pertussis doesn't seem to be related to parents' refusing to have their children vaccinated for fear of potential side effects. In California, pertussis rates are about the same in counties with high childhood vaccination rates and low ones. And the CDC reports that pertussis immunization rates have been stable or increasing since 1992," according to the *New York Times* in August 2010.

Even settling on a common definition of pertussis infection has been problematic for public-health authorities. An expert committee with the World Health Organization proposed a definition that "required 21 days of paroxysmal cough plus laboratory confirmation of pertussis in the subject or household contact," according to the journal *Pediatrics* in December 1999. "There are 2 problems with this definition," wrote the authors. "The first is that a substantial number of B pertussis infections in unvaccinated children are mild and would not meet the case definition. The second is that all pertussis vaccines tend to modify duration and severity of disease rather than completely preventing illness."

What? Substantial numbers of pertussis infections in unvaccinated children are mild? What else do we know about whooping cough infections in unvaccinated children? A study of a large number of unvaccinated children with laboratory-confirmed pertussis was published in *Pediatrics* in December 1997. "The age distribution of our patients with a peak in preschool children is typical for a primarily unvaccinated population. In contrast, widespread immunization results in a relative increase of cases in infants, adolescents, and adults," the authors reported.

The available evidence indicates that widespread use of the pertussis vaccine is changing the natural age at which whooping cough infections occur in our society. This finding coincides with CDC reports that more and more adults are suffering whooping cough infections, even as babies today are being infected at a younger age, an age at which they are considerably more vulnerable.

This age-spreading phenomenon has also been observed with other childhood infectious diseases for which mass vaccination has been undertaken, such as measles. The apparent desirable decline in the incidence of infection has been accompanied by an undesirable shift in measles infection to much younger, as well as much older, populations, for whom infection is far more dangerous.

Contrary to most media accounts and public-health announcements, the pertussis vaccine is incapable of preventing the spread of whooping cough. The CDC admits this fact on its Web site, but seems to forget about it in every discussion or press release about whooping cough: "The whole-cell vaccine for pertussis is protective only against clinical disease, not against infection. Therefore, even young, recently vaccinated children may serve as reservoirs and potential transmitters of infection."

The newer, acellular pertussis vaccines are even less effective than the older whole-cell vaccine referred to above, which had to be replaced because it was associated with "high fever, collapse/shock, convulsions, brain inflammation and permanent brain damage" in many children, according to Barbara Loe Fisher, director of the National Vaccine Information Center.

Does giving the shot to babies prevent the spread of pertussis infection in that population? Apparently not. "In fact, childhood disease predates the age at which children extensively socialize with each other and [pertussis infection] appears to commonly have as its source an adult, non or mildly symptomatic carrier," according to the *Journal of Clinical Investigation* in December 2005.

How about adverse reactions to the newer acellular pertussis vaccines? The CDC Web site tells us that one in 14,000 children receiving the acellular pertussis vaccine will suffer a seizure, one in every 1,000 will have nonstop crying for 3 hours or more, and 1 child in 16,000 will spike a fever of more than 105 degrees. Let's see, about 4 million babies are born each year, and each baby is recommended to receive pertussis injections at 2 months, 4 months, and 6 months of age—that's three pertussis shots in the first 6 months of life. Using the CDC's numbers, the pertussis shot is expected to cause 857 babies per year to have a seizure, about 12,000 to cry nonstop for 3 hours or more, and 750 to develop a high fever greater than 105 degrees. Are these alarming responses temporary, self-limiting, and benign? Are such vaccine-induced illnesses preferable to naturally acquired pertussis infection?

How about giving the shot to the rest of the population: Does that protect babies? "It is unknown whether immunizing adolescents and adults against pertussis will reduce the risk of transmission to infants," according to the makers of Adacel, a pertussis booster vaccine.

"The incidence and prevalence of pertussis in adults have increased in recent years. It has been shown that previously immunized adults and adolescents are the main sources of transmission of Bordetella pertussis," reported the *Chest Journal* in May 1999.

Let's review what we know about whooping cough and the vaccine. Death from a bout of whooping cough is rare; a well-nourished child typically comes through whooping cough just fine and ends up with lifetime immunity. Infants are the population most at risk of death from pertussis infection, and the infants who died in California in 2010 were too young in any case to receive the vaccine. The pertussis vaccine does not prevent infection but only modifies the symptoms. The vaccine is not capable of preventing transmission of pertussis infection to others, and previously vaccinated adults and adolescents are the primary source of the spread of pertussis. Many people who are fully vaccinated get full-blown cases of whooping cough. Outbreaks are on the rise even as vaccination coverage has climbed and remained high. Finally, widespread vaccination against pertussis has resulted in infants contracting whooping cough at a younger age and raised the ages at which adolescents and adults are becoming infected. In sum, based on 60-plus years of real-world outcomes, any reference to whooping cough as a "vaccine-preventable disease" is hopelessly inaccurate.

Scientific knowledge of the ways in which whooping cough is transmitted is anything but vague; vaccinated or not, people with an infection can infect others by direct contact. Despite a clear understanding of this fact, health authorities reflexively call for additional shots and blame the recurring pertussis outbreaks on unvaccinated people. Wouldn't it be great if parents were provided with tips on prevention that are based on actual science? Suppose health authorities educated the public about the fact that vaccination of everyone else cannot possibly protect babies under 3 months of age, and other measures must be taken?

In the midst of an officially declared whooping cough epidemic, the most appropriate response from our health authorities would seem to be a massive public outreach program that gives practical instructions on how to protect babies from whooping cough. The key is to avoid close contact between the baby and anyone suffering a pertussis infection. Close contact means touching and holding, as opposed to just being in the same room. Even so, preventing close contact is not easy, since the symptoms of pertussis infection for adolescents and adults may be no different than a lingering cold with a bad cough.

Whooping cough outbreaks have always been cyclical in nature. In the so-called post-vaccine era, this has not changed a bit. Widespread vaccination against pertussis has proven to be profoundly limited in reducing the spread of pertussis. These verifiable facts beg the question: What scientific basis do we have to support continued mass vaccination against pertussis? Where is the evidence that forcing more boosters on the populous each time there is an outbreak provides any benefit to any age group?

Author and clinician Archie Kalokerinos, M.D., has remarked that the historic importance of vaccines in public health is significantly overblown in the minds of public-health officials and the entire medical community. "Up to 90 percent of the total decline in the death rate of children between 1860–1965 because of whooping cough, scarlet fever, diphtheria, and measles occurred before the introduction of immunizations and antibiotics," he said.

"The definition of insanity is doing the same thing over and over again and expecting different results," said Albert Einstein.

Far be it for me to suggest that our public-health leaders are insane about the whooping cough issue. I'm just saying that doing more of the same thing we have been doing for more than 60 years and expecting the results to suddenly match the wishful thinking of our health leaders is ludicrous, counterproductive, and entirely disconnected from evidence-based public-health policy making.

Many parents who are choosing to not vaccinate their children have thoroughly researched the issue and are exercising their basic human right to make health-related decisions for their own children based on common sense. Reporters and public-health officials who haven't done their homework will undoubtedly continue making scientifically unsupported claims about vaccination and blame outbreaks on parents of unvaccinated kids as each outbreak rolls into town.

The vaccine controversy will likely be around for awhile, which is why it is so important to protect parents' right to voluntary informed consent and the inalienable right to refuse vaccination, or any other medical intervention, for their children.

Childhood Vaccination Against Sexually Transmitted Diseases: Protection For Whom?

You can die of the cure before you die of the illness.
Michael Landon

I attended elementary school way back in the early 1960s. Things were different back then—we had only one small black-and-white television in our entire house, and there were only three channels to choose from on TV. We children were also given only three vaccines that I recall, one smallpox and two polio vaccines—one live and one dead.

The Cold War was still simmering away, and duck-and-cover drills were a regular school routine to prepare us to survive a Russian nuclear bomb attack at a moment's notice. When the bell was rung, everyone crawled under a desk or crouched in a doorway with their eyes shut tight, except for the unlucky kid assigned to be the curtain monitor in each room, who first had to pull the curtains closed to "protect" the rest of us from the flash and blast of a nuclear explosion. As if.

Over the past 50 years, public-health officials have worked hard to pull the protection curtain over infectious disease, convinced that saving the health of our children requires strict adherence to an ever-busier vaccine schedule. Not only did the list of vaccines against childhood infectious disease expand to upwards of sixty doses in the interim, but babies and children are now also being vaccinated against sexually transmitted diseases (STD).

First came the hepatitis B vaccine. Vaccine enthusiasts touted this vaccine as the "first anticancer vaccine in history" because in theory, preventing chronic liver infection with the hepatitis B virus could prevent liver cancers in some chronic carriers.

The second vaccine for a sexually transmitted virus was the human papillomavirus (HPV) vaccine. Proponents of this vaccine also routinely call it an anticancer vaccine, against cervical cancer in women. We will consider the cancer prevention claims for the HPV vaccines in a moment, but first the hepatitis B vaccine.

This vaccine was developed to fight a viral disease of the liver encountered by adults practicing high-risk behaviors. Those at risk of hepatitis B infection include intravenous drug users who share needles, adults who have unprotected sex with multiple sex partners, and homeless alcoholics. Infection with this virus is essentially a self-inflicted disease, with the exception of medical workers who risk exposure to human blood in the course of their work.

So it was rather surprising when our health leaders decreed in 1991 that we should universally inject the new vaccine into every newborn baby in the United States. Our government agencies recommended that the initial vaccine be given within hours of birth, followed by two more doses by the age of 18 months, and a fourth booster shot at 11 or 12 years of age.

Was hepatitis B infection commonly found in newborns at that time? No. Was the vaccine ever tested for use in newborns? No. So why did the hepatitis B shot become the one vaccine all newborns receive in the hospital before they are even 48 hours old? "Because a vaccination strategy limited to high-risk individuals has failed," according to the product insert of one of the hepatitis B vaccines.

"Finding it difficult to vaccinate high risk groups with three doses of the vaccine, the government advisors decided the only way to control the problem was to vaccinate the entire population, starting at birth," explained vaccine researcher Sheri Tenpenny, D.O.

For a newborn baby, the chances of becoming infected with the hepatitis B virus are extremely small, requiring that the infant be either (a) born to an infected mother or (b) exposed to a blood product, such as a blood transfusion, that contains the virus. You may be forgiven for thinking that routinely screening the blood of all pregnant moms and then treating only the tiny number of children whose mothers are infected with hepatitis B would make more sense than vaccinating every single child in the nation, but that just proves you are not looking at the facts through the lens of a vaccine expert.

Vaccine experts seem unswervingly certain that vaccines are pretty much the complete answer to every public health issue imaginable. In the case of hepatitis B, it did not seem to matter that hepatitis B is an adult disease, is not highly contagious, and is not deadly for the vast majority of those who contract it; also, the incidence of infection was already in a historic decline. Vaccine promoters prevailed, and we began vaccinating every single one of the 4 million babies born in the United States each year with the hepatitis B shot while they were still in the hospital.

"The number of cases [in the United States] peaked in 1985 and has shown a continuous decline since that time," according to the *Guide to Clinical Preventive Services*. "Hepatitis B continues to decline in most states, primarily because of a decrease in the number of cases among injecting drug users and, to a lesser extent, among both homosexuals and heterosexuals of both sexes," reported the Centers for Disease Control (CDC) in 1996. The ongoing, long term decline in the incidence of hepatitis B infection continues to this day.

Suppose a person contracts hepatitis B. Just how dangerous is the illness? "Most patients with acute viral hepatitis experience a self-limited illness (one that runs a defined, limited course), and go on to recover completely," according to the Web site of the American Social Health Association.

"Approximately 20 percent of persons who contract hepatitis B will develop fever, abdominal tenderness and the telltale sign of the infection: jaundice. In this subset of patients, more than 95 percent recover fully and will be immune for life. This means of all persons who are both exposed to the virus and become measurably ill, only 5 percent have the potential to become chronic carriers of the hepatitis B infection," according to Dr. Tenpenny.

Hepatitis B is designated as a reportable disease, which means medical professionals are required to report cases seen in their offices. In 1991 the government tallied a total of 18,003 cases of hepatitis B. Since it is customary to assume that reported cases represent only 10 percent or so of the actual number, let us say there were 180,000 actual cases that year. Fully 95 percent of those infected, or 171,000 adults, would be expected to recover completely, with the benefit of immunity for life. That leaves 5 percent, or 9,000 people, with a chance of becoming chronic carriers of hepatitis B. Of that number, approximately 1 percent, a grand total of 90 individuals, would be expected to possibly go on to develop liver cancer.

This means that the decision to inject 4 million babies each year was apparently made in order to try and save about 90 people from potentially contracting liver cancer, people who display little regard for their own health in the first place, judging from their high-risk behaviors. The notion that injecting babies against hepatitis B can somehow protect those 90 adults is scientifically preposterous.

The drug companies each spent in the neighborhood of half a billion dollars to develop their hepatitis B vaccine, only to realize that their target demographic had no interest in getting the shot. I imagine it is pretty much impossible to convince junkies, homeless alcoholics, and prostitutes to go to a clinic and pay money for a shot that has a statistically insignificant potential for saving their livers from cancer some decades down the road. Could the real reason we decided to inject generations of children with this vaccine be to allow the drug companies to recoup their losses and make a profit on the shots?

The hepatitis B vaccine was the first genetically modified vaccine product in history to be approved by the U.S. Food and Drug Administration (FDA). A reasonable person might expect that the vaccine's safety would be studied very carefully before sticking it to all the babies, which serves to remind us that we should never make assumptions when it comes to vaccine research.

"In a group of studies, 1,636 doses of RECOMBIVAX HB were administered to 653 healthy infants and children (up to 10 years of age) who were monitored for 5 days after each dose," according to a product insert for Merck & Co. in 1993. They also stated "As with any vaccine, there is the possibility that broad use of the vaccine could reveal adverse reactions not observed in clinical trials."

Ya think? Come on, they observed the children for 5 whole days! What could possibly go wrong after a few more days, weeks, months, or years after injecting immunogenic, novel, foreign proteins deeply into the immune system? We can now answer that question by checking the published medical literature, since universal vaccination of newborns with the hepatitis B vaccine has been proceeding for 20 years.

Not surprisingly, more than a few health problems were missed by the researchers in their feeble 5-day observation trials. The list of vaccine-induced chronic neurological diseases and immune disorders in children and adults from administration of the hepatitis B vaccine is quite lengthy. The list includes lupus, arthritis—including polyarthritis and rheumatoid arthritis—Guillain Barre Syndrome, demyelinating disorders such as optic neuritis, Bell's Palsy, demyelinating neuropathy, transverse myelitis and multiple sclerosis, diabetes mellitus, chronic fatigue syndrome, vascular disorders, and convulsions, according to the National Vaccine Information Center (NVIC).

But wait, say the vaccine's advocates, these vaccine risks are as rare as hen's teeth, and besides, the risk of contracting hepatitis B is far greater! Oh, really?

"For most children, the risk of a serious vaccine reaction may be 100 times greater than the risk of hepatitis B…VAERS [the federal government's Vaccine Adverse Event Reporting System] contains 25,000 reports related to hepatitis B vaccine, about one-third of which were serious enough to lead to an emergency room visit, hospitalization, or death." This statement was made in testimony before a Congressional committee in June of 1999 by Jane Orient, M.D., then president of the Association of American Physicians and Surgeons.

Three years later, by the end of 2002, the number of adverse reactions following vaccination with the hepatitis B vaccine reported to VAERS had leaped upward. "In all, there were 38,600 reports to VAERS concerning adverse events and 753 reports of death, occurring at all ages, shortly after the administration of Hepatitis B vaccine alone or with other vaccines. The complications in 745 survivors were considered life threatening at some time. There were 14,476 Emergency Room visits, and 3,115 patients were hospitalized. 914 patients became disabled and 224 developed jaundice," according to pediatrician F. Edward Yazbak, M.D.

And a funny thing happened to the CDC's hepatitis B statistics once the vaccine was recommended for universal pediatric use. In an apparent attempt to justify its enormous campaign against hepatitis B, mathematical wizards from the CDC magically "updated" their numbers with a much higher and scarier "estimated incidence" of hepatitis B in the United States. Without citing any new scientific or epidemiological evidence, the number of Americans said to be suffering chronic hepatitis B infection suddenly shot up to 1 million, 5,000 of whom were now said to be dying from liver failure each year due to hepatitis B infection, and many others were developing carcinoma of the liver.

History tells us exactly what role the hepatitis B vaccine has played in the historic, ongoing decline of hepatitis B infection: complete and utter irrelevance. While it is true that the babies who were vaccinated 20 years ago are now young adults and are quite possibly engaging in high-risk behaviors that favor hepatitis B infection, alas, any ability of the vaccine to provide any immune response whatsoever is long gone by now. The junkies, prostitutes, and homeless alcoholics for whom the vaccine was originally formulated never did get the shot and still do not.

If your pediatrician tells you that the benefits of the hepatitis B vaccine far outweigh its risks, you might ask the doctor to cite the specific sources of his or her information. In all likelihood, the doctor is parroting wildly speculative and scientifically unsupported claims made by the CDC or else repeating advertising copy from drug company brochures. If the doctor would only invest a few minutes of his or her time consulting the peer-reviewed published medical literature for real-world outcomes assessments, the answer about the vaccine's safety would likely be quite the opposite.

What about the HPV vaccines? Merck Pharmaceutical's Gardasil was approved first, followed shortly by GlaxoSmithKline's Cervarix. In the beginning the three-shot series was promoted for girls only, but the HPV vaccine manufacturers were recently given the green light from the federal government to also push the shots on young boys. The benefit claimed for boys is the prevention of anal warts instead of cervical cancer—since boys have no cervix. But anal warts? Is it possible that our wise medical leaders were influenced by the drug companies in their sudden decision that protection against anal warts is an urgent matter in the health of American boys?

HPV vaccine promoters assert that the vaccine prevents cervical cancer in women by fighting infection with four different strains of HPV. Approximately 120 human papillomavirus strains have been identified so far, of which 12 are associated with—but do not by themselves cause—the development of cervical cancer much later in life. Since it will be another few decades before the girls currently receiving the shot reach the age at which women typically develop cervical cancer, any claims about preventing cancer are entirely premature.

Merck's study of the effectiveness of Gardasil was published in the *New England Journal of Medicine* in May 2007, claiming an astonishing 98 percent efficacy for preventing changes to the cervix—changes which the drug maker uses as a marker for potential cervical cancer. Merck's math department seemingly pulled its Gardasil statistics right out of a hat, because "when the researchers looked at negative cervical changes from any causes, they found that changes occurred in unvaccinated women at a rate of 1.5 events per 100 person-years, while vaccinated women had 1.3 events," wrote investigative journalist Jeanne Lenzer in *Discover Magazine* online in November 2011. That means the difference between the vaccinated and unvaccinated groups was two-tenths of 1 percent. Put another way, 500 young women need to be injected with the shots to reduce the number of events by 1. Recall that the term "event" here means not prevention of cancer, but prevention of precancer cellular change, a condition that normalizes for most women anyway.

"Most women who become infected with HPV are able to eradicate the virus and suffer no apparent long term consequences to their health...most infections by HPV are short-lived and not associated with cervical cancer," acknowledged the FDA in a policy statement in March 2003.

"Cervix cancer is rare in this country today," according to the American Cancer Society, "because most women get Pap tests that find it early or before it starts. Almost all women who have had sex will have HPV at some time, but very few women will get cervix cancer.... Most people will never know they have HPV. The infection usually doesn't last very long because your body is able to fight the infection. If the HPV doesn't go away, the virus may cause cervix cells to change and become precancer cells. Precancer cells are not cancer. Most cells with early precancer changes return to normal on their own."

And what about the minority of women whose cells do not return to normal on their own? "Cervical cancer occurs at an average age of 54; however, cervical intraepithelial neoplasia (or CIN), the precursor lesion to cervical cancer, most often occurs in much younger women. For a woman with CIN, her likelihood of survival is almost 100 percent with timely and appropriate treatment," according to the Web site for the CDC.

Just what are the risk factors for cervical cancer? From the CDC itself we learn that "the most important risk factor for developing cervical cancer, at least from the point of view of what we can do about it, is the failure to receive regular screening with a Pap smear."

Diane Harper, M.D., the principal investigator in the development of both of the HPV vaccines, has raised serious doubts about the justification for using HPV vaccines in the United States and other industrialized countries where regular screening with Pap smears has drastically reduced deaths from cervical cancer already.

"70 percent of all HPV infections resolve themselves without treatment within a year. Within two years, the number climbs to 90 percent. Of the remaining 10 percent of HPV infections, only half will develop into cervical cancer, which leaves little need for the vaccine," explained Dr. Harper at the Fourth International Public Conference on Vaccination in October 2009. Harper further stated that the incidence of cervical cancer has fallen to such low numbers in the United States already that "even if we get the vaccine and continue Pap screening, we will not lower the rate of cervical cancer in the U.S."

Dr. Harper also noted that we are vaccinating girls as young as 11 years old even though "There have been no efficacy trials in girls under 15 years.... There also is not enough evidence gathered on side effects to know that safety is not an issue."

"To date, 15,037 girls have officially reported adverse side effects from Gardasil to the U.S. Vaccine Adverse Event Reporting System (VAERS). These adverse reactions include Guilliane Barre, lupus, seizures, paralysis, blood clots, brain inflammation, and many others. The CDC acknowledges that there have been 44 reported deaths," said Harper.

It is significant that HPV vaccines are relative newcomers to the vaccine schedule, yet the VAERS data indicate they are associated with the highest incidence of induced abortions and stillbirths than any other vaccine in history. "The reported rate of serious adverse events is greater than the incidence rate of cervical cancer," summarized Dr. Harper.

More recent updates from the VAERS are even more alarming. As of April 2011 there were 95 deaths, and 21,634 reported adverse events following HPV vaccination. Whenever a VAERS report is made that includes hospitalization, life-threatening illness, permanent disability, or death, it is classified as serious. The number of serious events for the two HPV vaccines is double the number of serious events reported for any other recommended vaccine in the 7- to 18-year-old age group— even though the HPV vaccines are not the most widely used vaccines in that age group. If we apply the customary 10 percent rule to the number of reported adverse events, we are looking at shocking levels of serious health damage caused by the HPV vaccines.

To recap what we know about HPV, cervical cancer, and HPV vaccines: Most women will have HPV and never even know it. Cervical cancer develops only rarely. Regular Pap smears achieve early detection of precursor lesions of cervical cancer, and the vast majority of the pre-cancerous lesions go away on their own, in any case. The finding of cervical intraepithelial neoplasia (abnormal cells) is treatable, and the rate of survival is approximately 100 percent for women who receive this treatment. HPV vaccination does not eliminate the need for traditional cervical cancer screening, contrary to claims by many of the vaccine's promoters. HPV vaccines may or may not protect an individual against the targeted four strains of HPV, and it is not known how long this temporary immunity might last, although current estimates range from 4 to 6 years. No HPV vaccine has ever prevented a single incidence of cervical cancer. Ever.

By the way, if you are a woman already infected with one of the 4 HPV strains in the vaccine, your risk of developing precancerous cell change may increase by 44.6 percent and 32.5 percent, respectively, for Gardasil and Cervarix, just by having the vaccine injected into your body. This data was reported by the manufacturers and reported in an FDA review committee document in May 2006.

In light of all we know, you may be wondering how it is possible for our health authorities to continue advocating the use of either the hepatitis B vaccine or the HPV vaccines, much less both of them. You are not alone.

Interestingly, there is an inverse relationship between parents' education level and vaccination, according to the *American Journal of Public Health* in February 2007. Parents with the highest levels of education expose their children to the least number of vaccines, according to the study.

This news caused more than a bit of consternation and confusion among our public-health leaders, who have always assumed the opposite, that parents with more education would be more compliant with the vaccine schedule. One researcher, at a loss to explain the paradox, theorized that moms are probably just too darn busy these days with their careers and do not have time, or else they forgot, or else their decision to avoid vaccination stems from reading rants on the Internet written by knuckleheads and idiots.

A fourth possibility the poor fellow apparently found incomprehensible is that parents are doing their due diligence and researching the risks of the vaccines versus the risks of the diseases. They are making informed choices and expressing their fundamental human right of medical freedom to refuse medical interventions as they see fit. The number of parents who are opting out of vaccinating their children is rising as information becomes more available. One question in particular parents increasingly ask: Why in the heck are vaccine manufacturers granted blanket immunity for the death and disability directly caused by government-recommended vaccine products, year in and year out?

The American Medical Association (AMA) is quite annoyed these days that so many parents are doing their own investigations of mass vaccination and choosing to defy medical authority by just saying no. Rest assured that the AMA is not taking this insult lying down. The organization is busy trying to eliminate parents' vaccine exemption rights entirely, apparently in the belief that medical doctors are the only individuals smart enough to know what is good for our children. In its own words, "the AMA encourages state medical associations to seek removal of such exemptions in statutes requiring mandatory immunizations."

This reminds me of a story that highlights the shortcomings of accepting the idea that medical authorities know what is best for our children. Many readers may be old enough to remember the adorable March of Dimes poster girl from the 1950s, looking pathetic with her sad smile, standing in her leg braces and leaning on her two crutches. The back story about this little girl—never heard by most people—was related by author Eleanor McBean.

"Little Winifred Gardella had been treated for polio by medical doctors for two and a half years, and the best they could do was to release her as a hopeless cripple wearing crutches and leg braces—with no hope for the rest of her life. Her picture was used on the March of Dimes posters to jerk more donations from people….After she left the medical hospital, her mother took her to a drugless doctor, Dr. Lewis Robertson (chiropractor), who treated her with special drugless methods and had her well and walking in less than six months."

Parents need access to accurate and unbiased information about disease risk in order to make the best health care decisions for their child, and they need honest information about the potential risks and known limitations of every proposed medical intervention, including every vaccine and drug being recommended.

Dr. Joseph DeSoto of the National Institutes of Health explained this principle eloquently in an editorial in the Charleston Daily Mail. "Medical ethics require that patients have autonomy in their medical decisions, with informed consent. They have a right to know what they have, what the prognosis is, what the proposed treatment is, what the alternatives are, and what the possible side effects are prior to any treatment. Indeed, a patient has a right to say no, even if by refusing treatment they might die. I as a medical professional cannot overrule their decisions."

In elementary school back in my day, we were taught to never, ever trust Russian science because their so-called science was thoroughly corrupted by politics. We were instructed that scientific studies there were rigged and the reported outcomes were ideological in nature, having been decided upon ahead of time by political operatives. The scientist's apparent role was to fudge the experiments so the results would match the desired outcomes of the political leaders. To a young boy this was confusing, because didn't the Russian military have the ability to take out my town with a missile shot from halfway around the planet, and didn't that require some pretty sophisticated science?

At any rate, I am told that today in America we live in a modern, science-savvy society in which things are very different—meaning, I suppose, that our science is way better than the rigged Russian science was back in the day. Unfortunately, it appears that many often-repeated "facts" about diseases targeted by vaccines on the federal government's childhood vaccination schedule are fudged, as are many "facts" about the vaccines themselves.

At least we can congratulate ourselves that public-health decisions in the United States are not based on ideology. But then we must ask, what exactly are these decisions based upon, since the belief that children must be vaccinated against hepatitis B and HPV in order to be well is not supported in the scientific literature?

Ultimately, these STD shots actually do provide protection of a sort—just not the protection of anyone's health. It turns out that the only protection to be found in perpetuating the injection of hepatitis B and HPV vaccines into our babies and children is the protection of corporate profitability for the vaccine makers.

Flu Season Again

The joke's on them. One little hypodermic won't be enough.
Jodi Picoult

Don't you just love the changing of the seasons? Winter, spring, summer, flu… wait a minute, what day does flu season actually begin? I checked all the calendars in my house, but I could not find a single reference marking the first day of flu season.

After looking in vain through a few newspapers and abandoning a few Internet searches, I concluded nobody really knows for sure. Some sources pegged the opening at the first of September, others the first of October, and one Canadian newspaper was quite certain that flu season begins the first day of November. Even though there was no agreement about the season's opening date, all sources were agreed on two points: First, the flu season will be terrible this year, and, second, everyone should get a flu shot.

Public health leaders unanimously recommend getting annual flu shots. "The single best way to protect against the flu is to get vaccinated each year," according to the Centers for Disease Control (CDC). An increasing chorus of medical leaders is even calling for flu shots to be mandatory.

It seems that each year a new age group is added to the list of those who should get the shot. The list now includes pregnant women, not-so-pregnant women, tiny young babies, large old babies, children 6 months old to 6 years old, children 6 years old to 18 years old, the immune compromised, the ailing elderly, the not-so-ailing elderly, the middle-aged healthy, and the middle-aged not-so-healthy. About the only group that hasn't received a recommendation to get the flu shot is pregnant males over the age of 130.

We are repeatedly told that everyone "needs" the flu shot. Presumably, "need" in this context means "a flu shot is necessary to prevent infection with influenza." Indeed, helping people avoid a bout with the flu sounds like a great idea. How is that prevention thing working out so far?

"The vaccine doesn't work very well at all. Vaccines are being used as an ideological weapon. What you see every year as the flu is caused by 200 or 300 different agents with a vaccine against two of them. That is simply nonsense." That was the conclusion of lead author Thomas Jefferson, M.D., of the Cochrane Institute, reporting on an extensive meta-analysis of published medical research investigating annual flu shots.

The findings of another study about the flu shots published in the *Archives of Internal Medicine* in December 2008 can be summed up by my grandfather's old mathematics joke, Nothin' from nothin' leaves nothin'. Grandpa wasn't talking about the flu vaccine, but he might as well have been, because when the flu shot dose is cut in half, it apparently works just as well as a full dose. That's pretty cool; think of the money we could be saving, not to mention cutting in half people's exposure to the toxic cocktail that comes in each vaccine.

The half-dose study pretty well sums up the entire shot of logic in influenza vaccines: A dose of something that doesn't seem to work at all can be cut in half and work just as well. Or, to paraphrase Grandpa, start with nothing, take away half of it, and you get...nothing! But surely there must be some scientific basis for the massive flu-for-all extravaganza each year, right? Aren't there some published studies that prove flu shots work?

Well sure, the shots "work" in vaccine industry–sponsored studies, but only for subgroups of subpopulations in theoretical settings receiving a perfectly matched vaccine, and then only if the statistics are massaged to reach an arbitrary threshold of antibody titers in test tube samples of blood. As for preventing people from experiencing "the flu," or, more correctly, "flulike illness," it appears that the annual influenza vaccine rests on a foundation of faith, not science.

According to the authors of the Cochrane study, "Over 200 viruses cause influenza and influenza-like illness which produce the same symptoms (fever, headache, aches and pains, cough and runny noses). Without laboratory tests, doctors cannot tell the two illnesses apart. Both last for days and rarely lead to death or serious illness. At best, vaccines might be effective against only influenza A and B, which represent about 10 percent of all circulating viruses." But only when there's a good "match" of the predicted circulating influenza viruses in a given year.

Seasonal flu shots reportedly do have a modest effect reducing flu symptoms or days of work lost. How modest? At least 100 people need to be vaccinated to avoid one person getting influenza in an average year. In rare years when the three vaccine viruses in the shot actually match circulating viruses, vaccinating 100 people can save about three cases of influenza. But the authors warn that even this evidence of a tiny benefit may be optimistic, because their research included many studies produced by drug companies, and "company-sponsored influenza trials tend to produce results favorable to their products." No evidence could be found by the researchers that seasonal flu shots reduce complications such as pneumonia, nor was there any evidence the shots prevent person-to-person transmission of influenza.

To summarize the authors' findings, only 1 percent of vaccinated people are spared influenza infection, except in a really good year when it can go as high as 3 percent, but those estimates are likely quite optimistic because of investigator bias. Pretty amazing, isn't it? And our health leaders believe this to be "the single best way to protect against the flu."

I do not doubt that our health leaders sincerely believe that getting an annual flu shot saves lives and improves health. Perhaps the flu authorities have received a special inoculation that makes their minds immune to the overwhelming real-world data that fails to support claims of substantial benefit from annual flu shots. This is just one more example of public health policy being driven by consensus instead verifiable science. Evidence-based medicine regarding annual flu shots is just an important-sounding but empty phrase public health officials like to kick around.

If the goal of public health endeavors is to reduce the annual burden of seasonal respiratory disorders for individuals and the whole society, we have a tremendous opportunity to do so. But, first, our health leaders need to recognize that in the majority of cases when people are said to be suffering from "the flu," they are actually suffering from "flulike illness," not influenza. Flulike illness has nothing to do with influenza virus and cannot possibly be affected by any influenza vaccine, good match or bad. Second, our health leaders need to acknowledge the research showing an utter lack of unbiased, scientific evidence demonstrating that the shot is capable of anything greater than a statistically insignificant benefit for any age group.

If our public health leaders could take some time off from promoting vaccines against influenza and do a little research, they might discover that we already know about a reliable, inexpensive, readily available, and completely nontoxic substance that dramatically reduces influenza infection for every single age group the CDC wants to vaccinate. It is called vitamin D3.

Providing our bodies with sufficient vitamin D is emerging as a key factor in lowering the risk of influenza, influenza-like illness, and numerous debilitating and even fatal disorders. In the past few years the medical literature has produced volumes on the amazing properties of vitamin D, including the ability to prevent many cancers, mitigate heart disease, reduce high blood pressure, and reduce the incidence of type I diabetes, multiple sclerosis and depression, to name a few.

Vitamin D is more accurately described as a naturally occurring steroid hormone that increases the body's production of at least 200 antimicrobial peptides. "The 200 known antimicrobial peptides directly and rapidly destroy the cell walls of bacteria, fungi, and viruses, including the influenza virus, and play a key role in keeping the lungs free of infection," according to John Jacob Cannell, M.D., executive director of the Vitamin D Council.

The body makes its own vitamin D, but this requires sun exposure. It is perhaps no coincidence that the "flu season" occurs during the time of year people are more likely to stay indoors, resulting in diminished production of vitamin D.

According to Dr. Cannell, "A single, twenty-minute, full body exposure to summer sun will trigger the delivery of 20,000 units of vitamin D into the circulation of most people within 48 hours. Twenty thousand units, that's the single most important fact about vitamin D. Compare that to the 100 units you get from a glass of milk, or the several hundred daily units the U.S. government recommends as 'Adequate Intake.'"

Since increasing the body's natural production of vitamin D with exposure to sunlight is not always practical or possible, taking vitamin D3 supplements is a good idea. The Vitamin D Council makes the following recommendation on its Web site regarding supplementation with vitamin D3. "Take an average of 5,000 IU [international units] a day, year-round, if you have some sun exposure. If you have little, or no, sun exposure you will need to take at least 5,000 IU per day."

This year we are once again hearing about the supreme importance of vaccinating every single staff member, nurse, and doctor in senior-care facilities to protect the elderly from the flu. A separate Cochrane-sponsored study was done in Canada to try and verify the claim that the shot works. "What troubled us is that [shots] had no effect on laboratory-confirmed influenza," said lead author Roger Thomas, Ph.D., M.D. "What we were looking for is proof that influenza…is decreased. Didn't find it. We looked for proof that pneumonia is reduced. Didn't find it. We looked for proof deaths from pneumonia are reduced. Didn't find it."

Thirty years ago, when the government took up mass flu vaccination in earnest, influenza flu posed a health risk to very few people—namely, the frail elderly and those whose who are immune compromised. Today, the same people are still at risk for influenza. Despite a dramatic increase in the rate of vaccination, the death rate associated with influenza infection has remained a flat line. The flu shots simply cannot be shown to save any lives.

Decades ago, when mass vaccination against influenza was first deployed, a big fat assumption was made. It was assumed that artificially provoking the immune system into producing a temporary immunity to a few strains of laboratory influenza each year would make people and society as a whole healthier. Has the original assumption ever been tested using the time-honored scientific method at any point in the intervening decades? No. So the entire multibillion-dollar flu-shot apparatus is still operating on an assumption? Yes. And do we have name for science that is based on assumptions? Yes, we call it junk science.

Common sense and empirical evidence suggest it is more beneficial to our health for us to encounter wild microbes in the environment and mount an innate immune response free of medical intervention. Children with greater exposure to germs, dirt, and pet dander in their environment have been widely observed to have healthier immune responses throughout their lives when compared to children raised in relatively antiseptic environments.

"Getting the flu, whether type A or type B, was once a normal part of the human experience, an opportunity for both the developing and the mature human immune system to acquire cell-mediated immunity after confronting the ever-changing flu viruses that circulate around the globe every year," observed Barbara Loe Fisher, director of the National Vaccine Information Center.

In the words of pediatrician Larry Palevsky, M.D., "We all need to get sick occasionally to be well." Isn't it time we reallocate a small fraction of the money used to push flu shots to mount an authentic scientific study that compares health outcomes among vaccinated and nonvaccinated individuals?

The decision to receive an influenza vaccine is no trivial matter, considering what you get with each injection: Fragments of viral proteins known to trigger autoimmune responses, metals known to cause brain inflammation, and toxic chemicals for which the Environmental Protection Agency (EPA) registers no safe level of exposure because of irreparable harm to living cells. All these things are injected deeply into the body with each flu shot. A partial list of ingredients of a typical flu vaccine includes mercury (some vaccines pack a full 25-microgram dose, the rest have trace amounts), aluminum salts, formaldehyde, antibiotics, chicken egg protein, MSG, sucrose, polysorbate 80, and sodium phosphate, to name a few.

Pregnant mothers, children, and now babies are urged to get the flu shot, despite everything we know about the toxicity of mercury, even in trace amounts. Vaccine manufacturer's safety data sheets typically note that exposure in utero and in children can cause mild to severe mental retardation and mild to severe motor coordination impairment. Conveniently, no vaccine manufacturer may be held liable for death or damages caused by the government-recommended vaccines.

"If an individual has had 5 consecutive flu shots between 1970 and 1980, their chances of getting Alzheimer's disease is 10 times greater due to the accumulation of aluminum and mercury in the brain," stated Hugh Fudenburg, M.D., in a speech in 1997. Fudenburg is one of the world's leading immunologists and reportedly the thirteenth most quoted biologist of our times. More than a decade after Fudenburg made his remarks, flu shots still contain aluminum and mercury. The promotion of mass toxic exposure through the flu shot year after year is creating a tragic legacy of neurodegenerative, chronic illness in our society.

There is yet another major problem with flu shots that our public health leaders must face year after year: How do we safely dispose of the millions upon millions of vaccine doses left over from last year that nobody wanted? Flushing them down the toilet is illegal because the mercury and formaldehyde they contain are simply too toxic for the sewer system. Burying them in landfills doesn't work either, for the same reason. In the state of Utah, health officials literally throw caution (and mercury) to the wind and vaporize thousands of vaccine doses in incinerators each year. Talk about instantly creating a public health hazard for every living being downwind from the incinerators.

Dr. Jeanne Santoli, deputy director of the Immunization Services Division at the CDC, lamented, "It would have been great to use all the doses, because they don't protect anyone when they're not administered." She apparently has no idea how ironic her statement is, considering that the vaccines don't seem to protect anyone even when they are administered.

One proposed solution for the surplus is to not destroy the vaccines at all, but continue injecting people with them until they're used up. However, another vaccine expert, Dr. Walter Orenstein from Emory University, gets the credit for pointing out a major flaw with this plan. "You'd have to tell people next year that the vaccine they got could be inferior," he said. He makes a good point. Perpetuating a medical intervention that is inferior to one that has already proven to be of no use at all would seem to be a waste. A toxic waste.

Let's face it, the annual flu shot spectacular is big business. "The federal government has created a demand for vaccines by putting money on the table," noted Jose Rasco, an investment strategist at Merrill Lynch. "The profitability is back and the low margins are gone." Blind enthusiasm for flu shots is apparently quite contagious inside the government. Our wise congressional leaders doled out more than $1 billion of U.S. taxpayer money a couple of years ago to the grateful vaccine makers so they could upgrade their facilities and crank out even more flu shots and clever promotional campaigns.

Which brings us back to flu season scheduling. As long as our leaders insist on sticking to the whole flu-shot ritual, we should help them try and kick off the flu season properly. They probably feel pretty embarrassed that less than half the nation shows up for flu shots each year, including health professionals. The whole flu season marketing effort needs a complete makeover. Here are a few suggestions that might help fire up people's enthusiasm.

First of all, the kickoff for the season itself is completely vague. What day does it begin? We need a special day each year. The Official Flu Season Opening Day should be a holiday—fun, exciting, a celebration! Think parades, marching bands, baton twirlers, clowns, celebrity interviews, the whole bit. And we need some catchy slogans. "One for the money, two for the flu" is a step in the right direction, but obviously we need a national contest to come up with some hip messages. We also need to turn loose the pharmaceutical marketing boys so they can sign up flu season sponsors and plan promotions to last all the way to the last shot in the season closer. They could start with the obvious endorsements of products such as Official Flu Shoes and Official Fluffy Flu Facial Tissue. We'll need flu beer, flu chips, and flu season salsa. The ultimate goal should be an annual, massive, heavily promoted Barbeque For The Flu campaign.

Finally, we need an appropriate day for the season opener. I'm thinking the perfect match is Halloween. Hobgoblins, zombies and ghosts could easily help flu officials fan the flames of flu fear, especially since every single influenza vaccine already contains a witch's brew of chillingly creepy ingredients.

The Doctor of the Future

The man who says it can't be done should not interrupt the person doing it.
Chinese Proverb

Imagine a drug trial in which a group of people with high blood pressure were prescribed a new drug to lower blood pressure and instructed to take the drug one time only. Eight weeks later, all the people would have their blood pressure checked. Now, suppose that all the people were found to have lower blood pressure, with an average drop of 14 points for systolic blood pressure (top number) and a drop of 8 points for diastolic blood pressure (bottom number). Finally, suppose that not a single one of the people in the test group experienced a single adverse reaction.

A drug with this kind of remarkable ability and zero side effects sounds too good to be true, doesn't it? That is because it is too good to be true. No drug has ever existed that can make this claim. Don't get me wrong, dramatic results such as these are possible today, but not from a drug—or two, or even three.

"This procedure has the effect of not one, but two blood-pressure medications given in combination…And it seems to be adverse-event free. We saw no side effects and no problems," said George Bakris, M.D., leader of a study of 50 people with hypertension and spinal misalignment published in the *Journal of Human Hypertension* March 2007.

"When the statistician brought me the data, I actually didn't believe it. It was way too good to be true. The statistician said, 'I don't even believe it.' But we checked for everything, and there it was," says Dr. Bakris, director of the University of Chicago Hypertension Center. He was so impressed with the results he is planning much larger studies to verify the findings.

"Eight weeks after undergoing the procedure, 25 patients with early-stage high blood pressure had significantly lower blood pressure than 25 similar patients who underwent a sham chiropractic adjustment. Because patients can't feel the technique, they were unable to tell which group they were in," reported WebMD.

If a substantial, lasting reduction in blood pressure were actually possible by taking a new drug just once, I wonder how much money the drug company would charge for that pill? Ten thousand, twenty thousand dollars? It boggles the mind. Without a doubt, if a new drug came along that could reliably produce amazing results such as this, the news would make headlines around the world and blast the stock prices for that lucky drug company right into the stratosphere.

Meanwhile, back on planet Earth, we are not talking about a drug but a chiropractic adjustment. Chiropractic is best described as a science, philosophy, and art. It cannot be patented, nor can it be listed on the stock exchange and bought and sold for stockholder profits, all of which may explain why the medical community reacted to this remarkable hypertension study with yawning apathy or outright denial that these kinds of results are humanly possible, no matter the procedure.

Chiropractic has long been treated as the red-haired stepchild of the health profession, due in part to the millions of dollars spent by the American Medical Association (AMA) in the past "to contain and eliminate the chiropractic profession," in the actual words of its Committee on Quackery, which smeared chiropractic as an "unscientific cult." The now-defunct quackery committee was active several decades ago during the time AMA doctors were also appearing in paid magazine advertisements endorsing unfiltered cigarettes. AMA members at that time were officially forbidden to associate or consult with any chiropractors and were prohibited from referring patients to any doctor of chiropractic for any reason.

Finally, a formidable group of chiropractors, led by Chester Wilk, D.C., got fed up and in 1976 began a battle against the AMA that took 11 years. The lawsuit eventually reached all the way to the U.S. Supreme Court. The Supreme Court Justices let stand a lower court ruling that the AMA was indeed guilty of antitrust, engaging in an "unlawful conspiracy in restraint of trade," using "a lengthy, systematic, successful and unlawful boycott" intended to restrict collaboration between M.D.s and chiropractors and thereby eliminate chiropractic as a healing arts profession.

The AMA was fined and forced to formally recant decades of misinformation, disinformation, and name-calling. Nonetheless, those many years of lying and deceit had a lasting effect, and a sentiment still lingers among the medical community that chiropractic is less than scientific.

This is slowly changing as independent research bears out the chiropractic premise that adjustments reduce and eliminate interference to the innate recuperative powers of the human body. Much research is needed to fully understand how chiropractic adjustments are able to enhance a person's health globally. Some have even claimed that chiropractic's benefits cannot be said to exist until randomized clinical trials have been completed. Most chiropractors would welcome such trials, but the profession has yet to raise the many millions of dollars this research would require.

But this raises an important question: Should chiropractic be judged by a much higher standard than the standards of medical care? In other words, how many standard medical interventions have ever been carefully and properly raked over the coals of scientific scrutiny? Only about 15 percent of them, according to *The British Medical Journal* in June 1991. This means that eight or nine times out of ten, the drug therapies and surgeries prescribed by the average medical doctor have never been studied to see if they work.

Worse, only 1 percent of the articles in published medical journals are based on verifiable scientific research, according to David Eddy, M.D., Ph.D., the man who coined the term "evidence-based" medicine. This may help explain why well-intentioned medical intervention is now recognized as one of the major causes of preventable, premature death in this country.

"The problem is that we don't know what we are doing," Eddy said of allopathic medicine in *Business Week* in May 2006. Dr. Eddy describes our two-trillion-dollar-a-year medical system as operating with little or no evidence to support the notion that widely used medical interventions and procedures work any better than less invasive, less expensive alternatives.

But getting back to lower blood pressure, how is it possible for a specific chiropractic adjustment of the very top vertebral bone to result in lower blood pressure that stays lower? As the authors of the study, medical doctors every one, explain, "Minor misalignment of the Atlas vertebra can potentially injure, impair, compress and/or compromise brainstem neural pathways."

The brainstem neural pathways they speak of are the delicate nerve fibers in the neck responsible for communication between the brain and the organs of the body. The adjustment normalizes communication through the nerve pathways, allowing the body to restore healthy organ function, limited only by environmental, lifestyle, or genetic factors.

This is not to say that an adjustment of the Atlas bone is a "treatment" to reduce blood-pressure levels. The chiropractic adjustment does not treat any condition, whether a headache, neck ache, backache, sciatica, throat infection, ear infection, TMJ problem, sinus congestion, or asthma. Even so, people with these and many other conditions commonly find lasting, drug-free resolutions to their health challenges under chiropractic care.

Chiropractic is based on the principle that the body is a self-healing, self-developing organism guided by the body's own innate intelligence. This is the same unfathomable wisdom that organizes and directs growth from a single cell—resulting from the union of the male and female germ cells—into a fully developed human being in only 9 months. Innate wisdom does not stop there, but continues throughout life until the last breath.

Daily life provides us with stress that comes in three flavors: physical, emotional and chemical. To the extent that "stress" becomes "distress" in our bodies, disturbances may arise in the spinal nerve system, creating disturbances to the body's internal communication and a resultant loss of regulation over the body's interdependent life systems. Chiropractors call these disruptions to nerve flow one aspect of the vertebral subluxation complex, and the adjustment seeks to correct spinal function to reduce and eliminate such interference.

Although it is now possible to clinically measure positive changes in the body resulting from the adjustment, true measures of health go far beyond clinical indicators such as laboratory test results and the resolution of symptoms. Good health means physical, mental and social functioning at the highest levels.

Prophetic words attributed to Thomas Edison more than one hundred years ago seem well suited to the chiropractic profession, the world's largest drugless healing profession: "The doctor of the future will give no medicine, but will interest his patients in the care of the human frame, in diet and in the cause and prevention of disease."

Morning Sickness, Arbitrary Rules, and Old Wives' Tales

If nature had arranged that husbands and wives should have children alter- natively, there would never be more than three in a family.

Lawrence Housman

I heard it through the grapevine, "Jim and Allison are having a baby!" As if Jim had anything to do with producing the baby beyond the dubious "work" of getting the baby started. To be fair, Jim may actually be doing more work now, such as washing dishes and vacuuming the house, because Allison is busy in the bathroom throwing up.

"Morning sickness" is the customary and polite name for it, but when my wife, Nancy, was in the middle of that trying state of exis- tence, terms such as throw up, vomit, and barf seemed to carry more conviction and convey more gut feeling. The clinical title itself is pretty direct: Nausea and Vomiting of Pregnancy.

For Nancy and many millions of women, morning sickness might be more correctly called nonstop nausea. She bravely faced morning sickness and also midmorning, afternoon, late-afternoon, evening, and all-through-the-night sickness in the early stages of pregnancy with each of our two boys.

The obstetrician was cheerful, "Don't worry, after the third month it usually goes away!" as if Nancy would feel reassured hearing that the perpetual nausea, complete lack of rest, and no actual food digestion would continue for only two more months.

In my helpful husband role I did everything I could to lend a hand. These heroic efforts resulted in helping Nancy reduce her suffering by a factor of approximately zero. The big problem was that for Nancy, pregnancy altered her sense of smell and elevated her ability to perceive odor to that of a finicky bloodhound with jittery digestion.

One evening after slaving over a hot stove for more than an hour in the kitchen, I emerged victorious from the kitchen bearing a steaming bowl of delicious homemade soup. I grandly placed it on the table in front of Nancy.

"Ecch! You put celery in this soup, it's making me gag!"

"Honey, I put celery in this soup because you told me to put celery in the soup."

"Uggh, I can't stand the smell, I think I'm going to be sick!" and she staggered up from the table and hurtled down the hall to the bathroom.

Isn't growing a baby difficult enough without the added requirement of running to the bathroom to pray at the porcelain altar every 15 minutes or so?

I am wondering though, if it is a mistake to call this condition we do not understand a sickness. Question: Is a person "sick" who throws up their entire dinner if it turns out the turkey stuffing was teeming with, say, salmonella? No. Under such a circumstance, heavily heaving in a hurry is the healthiest possible response.

The innate ability to empty the stomach in an instant is a basic strategy the body has at its disposal to quickly eliminate toxins and also to alter the acid/base balance. Nausea and food aversions in early pregnancy will no doubt eventually prove to be just one more mystery of Mother Nature that we have been slow to figure out.

Many theories propose to explain why one-half to three-fourths of all pregnant women in the United States go through some version of prolonged queasy stomach misery, but so far we are only guessing as to the reasons why it happens. Is it a function of wildly fluctuating blood sugar? Is it the mother's body getting rid of minute toxins in food that are harmless to an adult but toxic to the sensitive developing system of a growing baby? Is it a deficiency of key nutrients?

Advice abounds for pregnant moms on how to reduce the frequency of gagging. This mainly centers on when to eat, what to eat, and what to avoid eating. I would like to nominate for the coveted "Most Astute Throw-Up Advice Ever" award for the following gem from an HMO: Avoid foods that trigger nausea.

The Latin word for vomiting is emesis. Emesis, according to my Dorland Medical Dictionary, "may be of gastric, systemic, nervous, or reflex origin, or due to irritation of vomiting center." Taken together these words mean that throw-up happens.

Other nauseating stuff happens during pregnancy, too. We were living in New York City at the time of Nancy's first pregnancy, and were denied midwife eligibility by our HMO because Nancy was 35 years old. We sat down and tried to reason with the highest administrative doctor willing to meet with us.

"Look Doc, only three people in Manhattan eat healthier than Nancy does. Her biological markers put her age 10 years younger than her chronological years, and she exercises religiously. She is in perfect health and wants to use a midwife, which we were told was available when we joined the HMO 2 years ago."

"She is 35, so she is too old."

"Okay. Suppose she was 34 the day the kid was conceived, but the next day was her birthday and she turned 35 that day?"

"In that case, there'd be no problem, she would have been 34 and still eligible."

"But she turns 35 one day later and the whole thing is off? Isn't that kind of arbitrary?"

"She would be ineligible because she would be older than the cut-off age. End of story. Do you have any more questions?"

"Okay, suppose the kid was conceived right at the stroke of midnight, just when she was more than 34, but not quite 35...?"

"Go away."

"But..."

"I'm leaving."

The doctor of utmost importance and wisdom then stood up and walked out of the room. The interview was apparently over.

We ended up paying out of pocket for a new plan: Nancy would deliver our son at a midwife center on the Upper East Side, at the time the largest freestanding midwife center in the United States.

Fast-forward several months after the interview with Dr. Arbitrary and the kid was 2 weeks past the due date. As an aside, isn't it amazing that only 4 percent of women have the baby on their due date? Anyway, we were told that if Nancy did not deliver the baby that very night, the midwives would have no choice but to refer us back to the HMO, meaning we would be transferred straight to the hospital two blocks away.

We talked to the midwife on the telephone and she recommended Nancy ingest some castor oil. We called the obstetrician and asked what she thought. "That won't work; using castor oil is just an old wives' tale." Thank the wise heavens for old wives' tales, because they apparently can be vessels of ancient wisdom. Later that same night we were on our way to the birthing center in a hurry, Nancy was having strong and increasingly frequent contractions as I drove. Poor kid, the castor oil tasted awful. It was mixed with something that smelled, looked, and tasted like nauseating minty yogurt. But it did seem to bring on the contractions in less than an hour.

Fast forward several hours, and it would only be a few minutes before Nancy would be required to transfer to the hospital, because according to the rules of the midwife center, more than 2 hours in the pushing stage is too long. That was when our little guy came flying out and we all cried. Nancy was my new hero forever.

Later that morning I fetched the car to drive us back to our apartment on the Far Upper West Side, also known as Upstate Manhattan, or Inwood. A traffic ticket was carefully tucked under the wiper blade of my car, which was sitting in the one parking space I was able to find in the middle of the night on the Upper East Side just 10 hours earlier. It was just one more unexpected expense of having a kid. But that was 22 years ago, and, in retrospect, the amount of the fine was nothing. Later, we would send the same kid to college.

And so the miraculous drama of couples producing children continues around the world at a brisk pace, and pregnant women continue to suddenly jump up, run out of the room, and head for the head. Nancy never did discover any surefire method to comfort her perpetually queasy stomach, but at the end of the third month of gestation, the nausea suddenly and happily subsided in both pregnancies.

Between seeking to understand the mysteries of Mother Nature, and coping with inflexible rules written and enforced by all-powerful White Male Doctors Robed in starched White Coats, having a baby is a lot of trouble for the new moms. Oh yeah, and it is also slightly inconvenient for the dads.

Midwives Save Lives

If we are to heal the planet, we must begin by healing birthing.
Agnes Sallet Von Tannenberg

America doesn't have too much trouble when it comes to starting babies, but for some reason we seem to drop the ball just when those babies are ready to make their grand entrance into the world. What is it about the American mode of delivering babies and our early care of the little ankle-biters that's killing us?

This question reared its ugly head again recently when America's newborn survival rates were compared with other modern, industrialized countries. How did we do? We tanked. At number 41, we lost out to Cuba. The good news? We are no worse than Croatia. The United States has a higher infant mortality than almost every other industrialized country in the world.

Let me hasten to assure you that the problem is not due to a lack of effort on the part of modern medicine. In fact, birthing babies has become big medical business in the United States, totaling more than $50 billion a year.

This situation raises a few questions. Is it possible our newborns are suffering because the medical profession is trying too hard? What problems are created for newborns when doctors try too hard? And just what is it those other countries whose babies are healthier than ours have that we are missing? The answer to that last question is that they have more midwives.

The name midwife means "with woman." Midwives have always been in charge of delivering babies, ever since the beginning of human existence, all the way up to about 150 years ago in the United States. That was when a small group of medical doctors decided to launch a war against midwifery, having unilaterally decided that medical doctors were better suited to the job than midwives.

What evidence did these scholarly gentlemen present to support the notion that they could do a better job? Evidence? Bah! They didn't need no stinking evidence! They had clout, they had money, they were men, and that was enough.

Recall that during this historical era, women still did not even have the right to vote.

No matter that birthing has always been an inherently low-risk, completely normal and natural human process for more than nine out of ten pregnancies. No matter that midwives and doulas have attended births since the beginning of time, passing on traditional wisdom to each new generation of women.

We can never underestimate the ability of a well-funded group of men to quickly move beyond mere facts when they decide to wipe out the competition. The strict moral code of wartime was immediately adopted by organized medicine: Never tell a lie unless it is absolutely convenient!

By 1920, the percentage of midwife-attended births had fallen from almost 100 percent to only 15 percent, and the heavy toll exacted by excluding midwives from the birthing room was already evident. One medical doctor lamented the inferior quality of U.S. births in 1921, "…the maternal death rate for our country was higher than that of every foreign country for which we have statistics, except that of Belgium and Chile."

Admit nothing, deny everything, and make counteraccusations! pretty well sums up the smear campaign used by medical politicians of the day to rid society of the "dirty, ignorant and superstitious" midwives. "We can get along very nicely without the midwife, whereas all are agreed that the physician is indispensable."

Not according to the authoritative, international study culminating in a book published in 1989, *Effective Care in Pregnancy and Childbirth*. The authors found little evidence to support the actions of those medical men who blustered and elbowed their way into the business of birthing babies. "You may be shocked to find what little evidence exists in support of most obstetrical practices...the evidence favors non-interventive management," wrote the authors.

"Doctors are not trained in physiological miraculous birth. They are needed as surgeons and high-risk specialists. They are highly trained in pathology," explained midwife and author Jan Tritten. "Using an obstetrician for normal birth is like using a pediatrician as a babysitter," said birthing specialist Marsden Wagner.

Numerous articles in the medical literature have reached similar conclusions. John Robbins wrote about one such study that compared an equally matched number of midwife-attended home births to hospital births.

"The study found that women birthing in hospitals were five times more likely to have high blood pressure during labor; nine times more likely to tear; three times more likely to hemorrhage; and three times more likely to undergo cesarean sections."

But don't outcome assessments show that all the interventions are justified to protect the babies, even if they are somewhat tough on the moms?

"The hospital-born babies were six times more likely to suffer fetal distress before birth; four times more likely to need assistance to start breathing; and four times more likely to develop infections," according to the study.

Hospital births are characterized by a relentless need to speed up and control the birthing process, resulting in numerous drug and surgical interventions that are costly, largely unnecessary, and frequently harmful.

"It [birthing] is not a medical event. There is almost no hope of a peaceful pregnancy and joyous birth within the medical system. Every woman needs and deserves the kind of nurturing and care a midwife provides," said Jan Tritten.

The overwhelming majority of births today happen inside hospitals, but only five or six generations ago, most babies were born at home. The laboring woman was typically attended by two other women, a midwife and a doula.

The decline in home birthing from virtually all births in the mid-1800s to just a tiny percentage today can be attributed to the power of organized medicine and its desire to place birthing in a medical context and environment.

Which brings me to my own birth. I was born in a hospital in Arlington, Virginia, way back in 1954. The story goes that I nearly made my grand entrance to this world in the back seat of my dad's 1948 Chrysler Windsor. Luckily, my mom managed to make it inside the hospital doors and lay down on the gurney before I made my sudden and very vocal debut onto the world stage rolling down the hallway.

Ah, yes, things were different back then. The nurses didn't even ask my parents about circumcision, they just whisked me off and whacked my wee-wee without asking. Those were the days of whack first and ask questions later, as automatic as slapping a baby on the behind.

I can imagine my mother's conversation with the nurse, "What's that little bloody bandage there on my baby?"

"Oh, that. It's from the circumcision, you know, we had to whack his wee-wee."

"You whacked his…but how come you did that?"

"Oh, it's nothing, we always do that to the boys."

"Oh! My poor baby!" And so on.

That was when the nurse bundled me away to a very sterile, very white, fluorescent-lit special room hilariously referred to as a nursery. The so-called nursery was actually a room full of little plastic boxes set atop rolling carts, each box holding a brand-spanking-new baby wrapped up in a little hospital blanket, each of us probably wondering what we did wrong to end up in the isolation ward. We boys, especially, having just had our most private parts whacked with a sharp instrument of torture, were particularly upset.

I am told that the nurses occasionally let us out for good behavior to see our moms, but only at feeding time. When feeding was over, they scooped us back up and hustled us right back to the starkly white detention room with the little plastic box beds.

I can only imagine what was going through my head at the time, "Where's my mama? Where's the warmth of her body and how come I can't hear that steady heartbeat I've been listening to my entire life so far?"

Things were definitely different back when I was born. Dads wouldn't even think of asking to come into the delivery room, much less expect to be invited inside. I am told we've come a long way since the dim, dark past of the mid-1950s.

For example, hospitals now allow dads into the delivery room to watch the birth. This allows them to experience the entire spectrum of feelings from sympathy to wonder and panic to sheer helplessness. Dads are known for their wise and helpful utterances in the delivery room, such as "ooh!" and "whoa!"

Also, these days circumcision has thankfully been relegated to the elective procedure list, now mostly recognized for what it always was, a cultural practice—although there are still plenty of foreskin-removal enthusiasts who persist in their claims that circumcision has medical and hygienic significance.

Speaking of medical significance and the plight of midwives, not long ago I was invited to be part of a community-based committee that was being formed to improve medical services out here in the back-country of San Diego County. Really important people were at the meeting, people from hospitals and clinics, people with power, rank and influence. And there was me, the token, symbolic, last-minute alternative, a nonmedical doctor for reliable comic relief.

The medical people mostly talked about the number of hospitals that have closed, forcing people to travel great distances to reach a hospital, the difficulty of finding funds to build new hospitals and clinics, and the terrible overcrowding inside the hospitals and clinics that remain in operation.

There was one idea floated by a member of the community at large during the meeting that made a lot of sense. What about creating free-standing birth centers out in the backcountry? Wouldn't that save moms from the anxiety of driving more than an hour to reach the hospital? Wouldn't birth centers save bunches of money and free up much-needed space in our overcrowded hospitals?

The idea was dismissed with zero discussion as though it was a bad joke, as if someone had nominated Santa Claus for president.

"Nope, can't be done," all heads shook as one. "No way, not profitable," they said with finality. End of discussion.

Not profitable? I left the meeting wondering how this was possible. I already knew for a fact that having a baby at a freestanding birth center costs, minimally, a third less than a hospital birth, and a home birth attended by a midwife costs about two-thirds less than a hospital birth.

Apparently, those important people at that meeting missed the article sitting on my desk at home in which Frank Oski, M.D., Director of the Department of Pediatrics at Johns Hopkins School of Medicine, reported, "$13 to $20 billion a year could be saved in health care costs by de-medicalizing childbirth, developing midwifery, and encouraging breastfeeding."

Granted, I'm not in the hospital business, but $20 billion a year in savings hardly sounds like chump change. How is it possible that saving chunks of money on that scale could not be considered profitable?

Midwives, of course, have been delivering babies since time immemorial. As author and family physician Sarah Buckley, M.D., has pointed out, "Women's bodies have their own wisdom, and a system of birth refined over 100,000 generations is not so easily overpowered."

But that does not stop ongoing efforts by erstwhile medical-birthing enthusiasts to snuff out natural birthing. Nonmedical births continue to be bashed by certain medical professional associations, who repeat the claim that home births are outmoded and dangerous and that hospital-based births are safer and produce better outcomes.

However, it only takes a brief review of the medical literature on this topic to grasp that there is a preponderance of evidence supporting just the opposite view. Midwife-attended births for low- to moderate-risk pregnancies (the majority of pregnancies), whether occurring in the home or in birthing centers, are proven to be as safe as hospital births. And because midwife-attended births in a nonmedical setting require dramatically fewer medical interventions, the already glowing record becomes even more stellar.

Medical interventions have an iatrogenic tendency, meaning each additional drug or procedure ordered by the doctor causes a new complication that not only interrupts the natural rhythm and progression of birth, but requires further intervention. This preventable cascade of medical interventions poses ever-increasing risks to both mom and baby.

A woman giving birth in a hospital is much more likely to have an epidural, a cesarean section (C-section), a vacuum extraction, or an episiotomy (the surgical cut to enlarge the vaginal opening), and she is more likely to receive pitocin (a synthetic hormone to induce labor or else kick labor into high gear), more likely to be catheterized, and almost guaranteed to be strapped down with an electronic fetal monitor so she can't move around or turn over during delivery.

Perhaps Ogden Nash was speaking of modern medical births when he opined, "Progress might have been all right once, but it's gone on too long."

Cordelia S. Hanna wrote of The National Birth Center Study, published in the *New England Journal of Medicine* in December 1989, "...about 15 percent of women who begin labor in a freestanding birth center require transfer to an acute care facility, while only 2 percent require emergency transfer. The others were mainly transferred for slow progress or because the woman requested anesthesia. The overall cesarean section rate was 4.4 percent."

Indeed, when first measured in 1965, the average hospital C-section rate across the United States was nearly as low as that of birthing centers, at 4.5 percent. But by 2004 the national hospital C-section rate had soared to 29 percent, nearly a third of all births. In some states such as New Jersey, the C-section rate exceeds 40 percent, and many individual hospitals report that a shocking 90 percent of all births end up with a C-section.

Perhaps this could be forgiven if a corresponding improvement in outcomes for mom and baby were in evidence, but that is not the case. The constant assurances from medical authorities that this upward trend reflects modern women choosing modern methods of birthing is pathetic passing of the blame, and the claim that high C-section rates reflect evidence-based medical practice is not supported in the medical literature.

According to the World Health Organization, the best outcomes for moms and babies occur with cesarean section rates of 5 to 10 percent, and rates above 15 percent are considered to do more harm than good.

The medical establishment's inability to explain our country's unforgivably high infant mortality leaves us no choice but to suspect every single medical intervention before, during, and immediately following birth as a potential contributor to preventable infant death.

The list of suspect interventions must include every medication, vitamin K shot, vaccine, and diagnostic procedure, especially those practices accepted as the current standard of medical care, including the epidurals, fetal monitoring, induced labors, C-sections, episiotomies, vacuum extractions, and catheterizations already mentioned, plus the multiple ultrasound scans routinely performed during pregnancy.

"Obstetricians and hospitals have found that high-intervention birth, warranted or not, is very profitable," said Tonya Jamois, president of the International Cesarean Awareness Network.

Finally I am able to understand why the idea of a low-tech, low-cost birthing facility for the backcountry was greeted with knee-jerk opposition by the medical representatives on the community board. Not-for-profit hospitals base decisions on profitability, and a freestanding birth center run by midwives would be just too low-intervention to be profitable. It is a tragic irony that the medical-birthing industry strives to maintain and increase layer upon layer of risk-laden and unnecessary interventions because it is so profitable, even though the available evidence tells us that freestanding birth centers would save the lives of many babies, not to mention a ton of money.

Carla Hartley, founder of Trust Birth, has pinpointed our dilemma, "We've put birth in the same category with illness and disease and it's never belonged there." In a hospital setting, birth is treated as an emergency, a life-threatening disease that requires high-risk interventions.

We need to think completely outside the box with birthing. Perhaps it is time to begin entirely separating uncomplicated births from the hospital, honoring birth as a normal physiological event. When it comes to giving birth, we need to get completely outside of the box we call a hospital, encourage births inside the home, and increase our use of freestanding birth centers.

The experience of bringing a child into the world is a universal and natural process. How can we plan and fund facilities, public education programs, and systems of transfer that reflect the requirements of natural, healthy birthing? How can we support the training and licensing of more midwives and expand the influence of that remarkable and timeless, but battered, profession?

We can no longer accept "oh, that's how we always do it" as a justification for continuing unwarranted medical interventions. To suggest that we must tolerate medical practices, procedures, and protocols because they are profitable just does not cut it anymore, literally.

Ultrasound During Pregnancy: Ultra-Unsound?

Today every invention is received with a cry of triumph
which soon turns into a cry of fear.

Bertolt Brecht

My favorite pregnancy ultrasound story came from a friend in New York City several years ago. After the helpful obstetric nurse completed a routine ultrasound scan on my friend's wife, the nurse checked her clipboard and said, "Oh, I see you two don't want to know the gender, that's fine." Halfway out the door she turned around and said, "Oh, by the way, are you going to want the circumcision?"

The first thing you notice about the use of diagnostic ultrasound during pregnancy in the United States is that virtually every woman has at least one ultrasound performed during her pregnancy. It has become symbolic of modern medical birthing. The second thing you notice, if you consult the American Medical Association (AMA), is that only a small handful of women should actually receive any ultrasound scans at all during pregnancy.

Officially, the AMA completely opposes routine ultrasound screening. In practice though, a list of the most common reasons ultrasound scans are performed is identical to the AMA's list of reasons for *not* using an ultrasound. According to the AMA, attempting to answer the following questions using ultrasound scans does not justify the risk of exposure to ultrasound radiation: Is it a boy or a girl? What is the age and size of the baby? Is it a multiple pregnancy? What is the position of the baby in the womb? As my wife, Nancy, commented, "Those are the exact reasons they gave me when I was told to go get an ultrasound during my pregnancies!"

Prenatal ultrasound is so common that many people believe ultrasounds are absolutely necessary in order to ensure a healthy pregnancy. How did ultrasound scans become absolutely routine, despite serious cautions from the AMA? Could it be that the doctors, nurses, and technicians are all trained to use the latest expensive medical technology, allowing the hands-on skills once passed down through generations of midwives and doctors to pass into oblivion?

The American Institute of Ultrasound in Medicine (AIUM) maintains that no negative biological effects on pregnant women have ever been confirmed from the use of ultrasound scans. Of course, if you never look for something, you'll never find it. The makers of costly medical technology have zero financial incentive to verify the bad news suggested by the few independent studies that actually have been done.

And what about the health of the babies who are exposed to ultrasound radiation during gestation, many of them repeatedly? Substantial evidence is accumulating that suggests ultrasound exposure has a massive potential to harm a growing fetus.

"Studies on humans exposed to ultrasound have shown possible adverse effects, including premature ovulation, pre-term labor or miscarriage, low birth weight, poorer condition at birth, dyslexia, delayed speech development, and less right-handedness, a factor which in some circumstances can be a marker of damage to the developing brain," according to Sarah Buckley, M.D., author and family practitioner in Australia.

"Animal experiments have demonstrated lung, kidney, and other organ injuries due to nonthermal effects of ultrasound exposure," wrote Dev Maulik in his book *Doppler Ultrasound in Obstetrics and Gynecology*.

"Nor should it be forgotten that in the monkey studies the ultrasound babies sat or lay around the bottom of the cage, whereas the little control monkeys were up to the usual monkey tricks. Long-term follow up of the monkeys has not been reported," said British author Beverley Lawrence Beech.

"A series of studies compared the effects on birth outcomes of routine ultrasound screening versus the selective use of the scans. One of these randomized trials, published in the *New England Journal of Medicine* September 1993 involved 15,151 pregnant women. The last sentence of the article is unequivocal: 'Whatever the explanation proposed for its lack of effect, the findings of this study clearly indicate that ultrasound screening does not improve perinatal outcome in current U.S. practice,'" according to Michael Odent, M.D., founder of the Primal Health Research Centre in England.

What do we know about the immediate biological effects that occur when ultrasound radiation interacts with living human tissue? The focused, high-energy beam causes two distinct effects in the body, both of which generate heat. The first is a local temperature rise of about 2° Fahrenheit in the radiated tissue. It is a widely presumed that this small rise in temperature in and of itself is insignificant.

The second is cavitation, a process whereby small pockets of gas present in human tissue vibrate rapidly and then collapse. Temperatures in the gas are said to reach many thousands of degrees Celsius. This alters normal human chemistry in the vicinity of the generated heat. A number of abnormal, potentially toxic chemicals are produced within the cells in this way. The effects of this toxicity on the rapidly dividing cells of a growing baby are currently not known because they have not been studied.

Routine ultrasounds are notorious for a high percentage of false-positive findings that scare the heck out of pregnant moms. This causes anxiety, further unnecessary and invasive testing and interventions, increased cesarean births, and fewer babies carried full term.

Babies exposed to ultrasound energy seem to "hear" intense sound, even though the frequency of ultrasound waves is outside the auditory range of humans. Researchers believe that the rapid vibration of the tiny, developing hearing structures caused by the ultrasound energy produces the effect of hearing. According to Mayo Foundation researcher Mostafa Fatemi, Ph.D., babies experience ultrasound as an intensely loud sound "equivalent to the level of sound produced by an approaching subway train." Having lived in New York City for several years when I was younger, I can vividly appreciate that description.

Then there is the very popular phenomenon of what I call "recreational ultrasound," the three- and four-dimensional ultrasound scans done purely for entertainment value to create prebirth baby pictures and videos. These devices bounce multiple beams of ultrasound radiation into the womb, whose echoes are processed to create an image of the baby. There is no clinical benefit for using this technology, period. The marketers and purveyors of recreational ultrasound call it "elective ultrasound." The U.S. Food and Drug Administration (FDA) calls it "an unapproved use of a medical device," but to date the agency has done nothing to stop the practice. (This may be due to the fact that FDA staff is kept too busy shutting down raw milk coops, and vitamin companies who have the audacity to suggest on their product labels that food supplements can enhance human health.)

Expectant couples can walk into an ultrasound depot, with no medical referral necessary, and fork over about a hundred and fifty bucks to watch their unborn baby on a large television screen flail tiny arms and legs while twisting its little head back and forth. "Look Daddy, the baby is smiling and waving at you on TV!" Parents no doubt imagine their baby is twisting and flexing arms, hands, and torso and opening and closing its mouth during the ultrasound videotaping because the baby wants to say hi to Mommy and Daddy. Research however, tells us that these active motions begin only when the ultrasound beam is switched on, and the squirming motion represents the baby's desperate attempts to escape the penetrating radiation.

Some readers may be old enough to remember another unregulated medical device from the past, those x-ray shoe-fitting machines in shoe stores that allowed you to see your foot inside the shoe. Kids loved playing with those x-ray fluoroscopes while their moms were busy buying shoes, taking turns putting in feet, hands, and elbows. Luckily, the opening at the bottom of the gizmo was too small to fit in a head. Who knew the little box was emitting a steady stream of ionizing x rays into the children's bodies as they played, or that the clerks in those stores were absorbing enormous quantities of scatter radiation day after day? The machines were not discarded until decades after the radiation dangers were well recognized and discussed.

The Bureau of Radiological Health describes diagnostic ultrasound as "non-ionizing radiation." Ultrasound was first developed as a military tool to detect enemy submarines in World War II and then became a powerful medical imaging tool. It has now evolved as a political tool, championed by antiabortion groups for its ability to portray graphic images of very early human life inside the womb. This may help explain why we have not seen any serious attempts to date to create sensible federal regulations that would curtail frivolous ultrasound scans.

Consider the words of former president George W. Bush, quoted in the *Toledo Blade*: "Today, through sonograms and other technology, we can clearly—see clearly that unborn children are members of the human family, as well. They reflect our image, and they were created in God's own image." With friends in high places, the perpetuation of zero to lax federal regulations over recreational ultrasound is not really surprising.

The proliferation of unnecessary ultrasound exposure begins to sound like déjà vu all over again, a tragic replay of the history of medical x rays. For fifty years, medical doctors enthusiastically endorsed routine use of x rays during pregnancy. The x-ray habit persisted even as the cumulative, carcinogenic effects of x-ray exposure became well recognized.

We now have the experience of about forty years of the use of diagnostic ultrasound in obstetric practice and still we wait for long-term safety studies. All this time we have repeatedly heard from the ultrasound enthusiasts in the birthing industry that ultrasound is a benign technology, safe for routine use, and is not even a problem when used recreationally, in spite of the much greater ultrasound exposure. None of these safety claims is supported in the scientific literature.

"Although we now have sufficient scientific data to be able to say that routine prenatal ultrasound scanning has no effectiveness and may very well carry risks, it would be naive to think that routine use will not continue," wrote Marsden Wagner, M.D., international authority on childbirth.

Practitioners have widely abandoned the old-fashioned method of using skilled hands and stethoscopes to conduct prenatal exams. We have instead come to rely on ultrasound scans, despite our ignorance of the myriad health problems this practice may be causing our newborns. Our babies and children are not only more medicated and vaccinated than any other youngsters on the planet, but more radiated with ultrasound too. In the process of "modernizing" and "medicalizing" pregnancy and birth, we seem to have lost the ability to perform completely safe and reliable hands-on prenatal health assessments. This may be a classic case of throwing out the baby with the bathwater.

PreMedicine for PreProblems

Prediction is very difficult, especially if it's about the future.
Niels Bohr

The pharmaceutical companies have done it again: They have proven the depth of their genuine concern for the health of our entire citizenry. They are so concerned, they are "preconcerned." And what does this mean? It means that scientists working for the pharmaceutical companies believe they have discovered a key concept about our health. Hundreds of millions of us have been walking around thinking we were doing pretty well healthwise, but actually we are all in the early stages of chronic presickness. That's right, it turns out that the human condition is really just a temporary precondition before we get debilitating diseases.

Now, before this worrisome news triggers any preanxiety attacks or predepression mood swings, please hold on, because help is on the way. But first let us review the prefacts.

120

Having healthy clinical signs and passing all the diagnostic tests with flying colors means nothing at all anymore. In the old days the EKGs, CBCs, EEGs, x rays, MRIs, CAT scans, PET scans, Paps, and PSATs were trusted indicators of an individual's health condition, but no longer. This does not mean doctors will henceforth cease ordering all those tests, it just means the results will be duly noted and fully ignored.

The first signs of the coming wave of presickness emerged a few years ago with a smattering of diagnoses being charted for "prehypertension." With prehypertension, the heart sounds good, the cardio tests are good and everything else about the person's health seems to be fine. Fine, that is, unless you have been specially trained to spot the subtle signs of prehypertension, such as a patient who has a pulse or wears shoes.

A related but also widely overlooked presickness that affects virtually the entire population of the United States is pre-high cholesterol. If you have "good" cholesterol numbers, don't be fooled. If your current M.D. tells you your blood test results are "normal," you need to switch to a doctor who knows what's what. Normal means only one thing: pre-abnormal.

But now, thanks to all of the hard work and sacrifices of Big Pharma and its doctors, scientists, and government regulatory hand puppets, the solution is finally at hand with the realization that we are all born to be sick. You know all those unrealized potential health problems everyone thinks they might develop after hearing about them on television ads? It turns out we are all in the initial stages of each and every one of them. If you are well, you are presick. If you are sick, well, you're just sick. Got it?

I wonder why it took researchers so long to uncover the simple truth here. In order to affix the "pre" to prehypertension, pre–high cholesterol and predepression, all that is needed is—get ready—a diagnosis! You know what I'm talking about, an insurance billing code. It's for the drugs. One pill each day for the rest of your life for each preailment you might possibly one day be at risk of potentially having, maybe. But don't worry, these drugs have all received the coveted FDA Seal of Preapproval.

Are you surprised that drug-company-funded scientists were able to come up with such a refreshingly ingenious and original idea? Not me, I have come to expect nothing less from the laboratories of our fine drug houses.

The amazing part about all of this presickness is that the drugs needed to treat all these scary preproblems have been right under our nose the whole time. This means we won't have to wait for years while the FDA wastes precious time mulling over the silly problem of drug side effects and safety issues.

That is because the very same drugs that doctors have been prescribing to treat actual hypertension will work just fine for prehypertension. Likewise, pre–high cholesterol can be treated with the actual high-cholesterol drugs, predepression can be treated with real depression antidepressants, and so on. Preheadache, preheartburn, preconstipation, preattention deficit disorder—the list of preproblems stretches on seemingly forever.

I wonder if the drug companies have realized they are sitting on a veritable gold mine? Ha ha, I'm only joking, of course they have. Once people can be made aware of the entire panoply of preproblems that are possible through additional advertising, all the new preprescriptions will be flying off the pharmacy shelves faster than you can say pill popper. Then, at the point when presickness begins tapering off and actual health problems begin showing up, the only thing doctors need to do is ramp up the dosage using the same meds. Brilliant.

National health leaders are eagerly preparing preplans. They have concluded that the massive precomplaints facing our society are so daunting and so extensive that it requires massive presickness preparatory education. Qualified doctors will soon begin receiving predisease training at special preschools. Once doctors have been carefully pretrained to prediagnose prediseases, they can properly prescribe premedications. Of course, they will also need to know when to refer out for presurgery.

I guess the only question left is, who is going to prepay for all of this? Just kidding! We already know the answer to that one.

Drugging Our Children

It is easy to get a thousand prescriptions, but hard to get one single remedy.

Chinese Proverb

The prescribing of powerful psychoactive drugs as the primary strategy for solving social behavior problems has become standard medical procedure in America. Can anyone explain the puzzling paradox that stimulant drugs stimulate adults and yet they seem to calm children? No, not the drug makers, and certainly not the doctors doing all the prescribing. I wonder what else we don't know about these drugs?

I also wonder who originally had the cruel idea of placing 30 or more children in school classrooms day after day, week after week, with only one or maybe two adults in charge? If you have ever observed an elementary classroom in session, you know for certain that the majority of the students, especially the boys, are just barely able to keep a lid on their natural instincts. Instincts include leaping onto chairs and desks, leaping off chairs and desks, random vocalizing at 120 decibels, and hurling erasers, tennis shoes, apple cores, and insults at students across the classroom.

I come from a family of schoolteachers. My mother's teaching career spanned 30 years, prior to the era of treating the difficult behavior of children with chemical straightjackets. But other family members and friends who are teachers tell me they know just how effectively Schedule II narcotics work to calm down hyperenergized boys and the occasional girl. Unfortunately, the problem kids who are given the drugs are also given the very sticky label of Attention Deficit Disorder (ADD) or Attention Deficit Hyperactivity Disorder (ADHD). I call them sticky labels because they are so easy to slap on and so difficult for the kid to remove later in life.

Today's overworked, underpaid teachers, who are expected to teach and inspire an overcrowded classroom of kids hyped up on video games, television, sugar, and junk food filled with neuroexcitatory artificial flavoring and colors, understand just how well drugging works. Dosing a handful of thoroughly out-of-control boys with narcotic stimulants can prevent the whole class from erupting into hopeless chaos; chaos that may erupt spontaneously at any moment.

Lately I've been wondering about the widespread use of pharmaceuticals as a solution for problems in the school setting. Troubled by the thought that there may be a slight downside to keeping 4 million American children amped up on powerful prescription medication all day long every day, I sought the opinion of the highest authority in the land, the American Psychiatric Association (APA). Here's what our country's top psychiatric minds have to say on the subject of drugging our children, according to Jason Young, the APA's communications manager: "Yes, there is overprescribing, but there is also underprescribing." I am not making this up.

Detecting considerable confusion in the APA's statement, I realized the organization could use our help clearing up this issue. It has come to my attention that some readers of this very essay may themselves be having trouble paying attention. Therefore, as a vital public service that may be of help to the entire community, let us endeavor to find out just how many of us have the APA's dreaded ADHD "disease" and settle the overprescribing/underprescribing riddle.

Testing ourselves will help us to discover who really needs professional help—meaning, of course, which ones of us need powerful mind-altering drugs on a daily basis. Ready? No, of course you're not ready, because when was the last time you were asked to take a test in the middle of an article about ADHD? But just relax and get comfortable, we'll be done before you can say, "Hey, anybody seen my keys?"

Okay, remain calm, be honest with yourself, and don't cheat by looking at your neighbor's answers. Answer each question with yes or no. There are no "maybes" or "sometimes" in this test. By the way, if you do happen to answer yes to more than two questions, it only means that you have been formally diagnosed with a major social/behavioral disorder. But don't be nervous.

Here we go, yes or no: Do you fail to pay close attention to details, or make careless mistakes? Are you easily distracted by irrelevant sights and sounds? Do you have trouble following instructions carefully? Do you have trouble listening when spoken to directly? Is your desk a big mess? Do you lose or forget things you need, such as your pencil, your keys, or your cell phone? Do you skip from one uncompleted activity to another?

See? Making a diagnosis based on a list of behaviors is not rocket science, in fact, it is not science at all! It is called psychiatry. Anyway, I had to answer yes to most of the questions. I wonder which pills I need?

The test questions above are a sample of actual questions asked by real medical doctors to diagnose ADD or ADHD, right from the source: the *Diagnostic and Statistical Manual, Fourth Edition, Text Revision*. No brain scan, blood test, or any other kind of objective biological or physiological testing is available to make an ADHD diagnosis. See how easily children can acquire labels and be placed on daily narcotics?

"ADHD doesn't exist—it is not a physical abnormality, and as such bears no risk of causing physical injury or death as does every drug used in its treatment," said Fred Baughman Jr., M.D., author of the book, *The ADHD Fraud—How Psychiatry Makes Patients of Normal Children*. He rejects the idea that millions of children have something that can accurately be called a disease, and they certainly do not suffer from a deficiency of powerful psychoactive drugs buzzing around in their central nervous system.

The late pediatrician and author Lendon Smith, M.D., agreed: "It is too bad that psychiatrists have failed to recognize that if a stimulant acts as a calming agent, then they must shore up the flagging enzyme that is under-producing." He refers here to the production of norepinephrine and the ability of the brain to disregard unimportant stimuli. Dr. Smith found during more than 55 years of practice that supplementation with magnesium, calcium, vitamin B6, essential fatty acids, and avoidance of milk helped many overactive children to remain calm.

A 9-year-old boy we'll call Eric was diagnosed with ADHD by his family's medical doctor and was promptly prescribed stimulant drugs to control his behavior. His mother, dissatisfied with the medical diagnosis, brought him to me, a chiropractor. In my examination I quickly discovered a key underlying physical problem apparently missed by the medical doctor: Eric had a perpetual need to relieve intestinal distress caused by chronic production of flatus. In other words, Eric had difficulty sitting still and paying attention because of his digestive system; he had so much intestinal gas he was constantly focused on trying to prevent external combustion.

As you may recall, elementary school etiquette reckons the passing of gas to be entirely unacceptable behavior, yet outrageously hilarious every time it does occur. With the exception of the far corners of the playground outside, control of this particular bodily function is implicitly expected at school, and violators are ruthlessly ridiculed. Even when kids are outside, they must be aware of which way the wind is blowing to avoid massive and cruel teasing.

Antisocial behaviors and inattentiveness can have numerous underlying causes. In Eric's case, a short course of chiropractic adjustments reduced vertebral subluxation in his spine, and his problem vanished. With improved spinal neurological function came improved function of his digestive tract and a restored ability to concentrate in class.

Other challenges that can cause behavioral problems include food allergies, nutritional deficiencies, hearing problems, problems with vision, hypoglycemia, thyroid problems, and even mercury and lead toxicity, to name a few. What is the likelihood that many of the more than 4 million children currently taking stimulant medication to control ADHD behaviors have underlying physiological problems undetected by their medical doctor? Many experts believe the number to be enormous.

Another question asked by parents is this: Does giving stimulant drugs to these kids ultimately improve their lives by helping them stay focused and allow them to get ahead in school? No one knows, because no long-term, follow-up studies have ever been conducted to find out how these kids fare later, compared to children who are not drugged.

And just how safe are these drugs anyway? "An FDA report from April 2004 noted 51 U.S. deaths among patients taking ADHD medicines. Other reports described high blood pressure, chest pain, heart attacks, strokes, irregular heartbeats and fainting," wrote Lisa Richwine for Reuters in February 2006. "Drugs taken by millions for attention deficit hyperactivity disorder should come with strong warnings that they may raise some patients' risk of heart problems, a U.S. advisory panel said on Thursday," reported Richwine, detailing an FDA advisory panel's recommendation for a black-box warning. The FDA ignored the panel's recommendations, and, sadly, no warning was added to the drug packaging.

The list of common side effects of the stimulants includes feeling restless, difficulty sleeping, loss of appetite, headaches, irritability, upset stomach, depression, dizziness, and tics. Stimulants are also reported to trigger or exacerbate symptoms of psychiatric disorders such as paranoia, depression, agitation, hostility and anger, disinhibition, hypomania and mania, aggression, and anxiety, according to Peter Breggin, M.D., author of the book, *Talking Back To Ritalin*. Breggin argues that parents, teachers, and even doctors have fallen for the marketing tactics used by the drug companies. "Drug companies have targeted children as a big market likely to boost profits and children are suffering as a result," said Breggin.

Dr. Breggin claims that ADHD drugs can bring on the symptoms they are supposed to treat, such as hyperactivity, inattention, and impulsivity, and this leads to a vicious circle of higher medication doses, along with an increased danger to the child's health and well-being.

The pharmacologic action of many ADHD drugs is nearly identical to cocaine, but the effect on brain receptor sites can be even more potent. This perhaps explains why a million people not under the care of a medical doctor regularly crush up these same pills and snort the powder to get high at college parties and the like. The illicit or recreational use of ADHD drugs accounts for fully 20 percent of all consumption of the drugs in the United States. Interestingly, unlike other Schedule II narcotics such as amphetamines and cocaine, the ADHD stimulants used illicitly are all manufactured by the big drug companies—there are no illegal laboratories cranking out knock-off versions for sale. The Drug Enforcement Agency ranks this class of drugs near the top of the list of stolen drugs.

So, how did you do on the test? Got ADHD? Yeah, me too, I guess—but I think I will skip the drugs and just work harder on concentrating. You still can't find your car keys? No, I haven't seen them, but after you find yours, maybe you could help me look for mine?

Coming Soon to a Child Near You:
The War On Cholesterol

Doctors are men who prescribe medicines of which they know little, to cure diseases of which they know less, in human beings of whom they know nothing.

Voltaire

The American Academy of Pediatrics (AAP) recently announced guidelines to tackle cardiovascular disease in children by screening kids as young as 2 years old for cholesterol levels. If the cholesterol numbers are too high, the new AAP plan advises doctors to first promote weight loss and increased physical activity, and to provide nutritional counseling. Secondly, the recommendation is to prescribe cholesterol-lowering drugs, called statins.

Focusing on healthy hearts for young people is a great idea. Heart disease is one of the leading killers in our nation, yet it is largely preventable, a lifestyle-induced disease. The AAP's shift in thinking

appears to be a welcome and significant change for the pediatric professional trade association. The suggestion that children can achieve
better health through better nutrition seems to be a 180-degree about
face for the AAP, which has for decades scorned and scolded parents for
choosing to improve their child's health and behavior using special diets
such as the Feingold diet.

The Feingold program is concerned primarily with total avoidance
of artificial sweeteners, colors, and chemical flavoring, and the exclusion of certain salicylate-containing foods. For 35 years the AAP dismissed the Feingold diet as worthless quackery, while promoting
psychoactive drugs and narcotic stimulants as a superior, scientific strategy for modifying child behavior. Did the leaders at the AAP all those
years consider parents to be too simpleminded to know whether or not
their children experienced a shift in hyperactive behavior or lost weight
after switching to a specialized food plan?

It is to be hoped that the AAP's decision to pursue the improvement
of kids' heart health signals a departure in standard pediatric weight-
loss strategies. In the past these strategies have pretty much consisted of
prescribing stimulant drugs to curb appetite along with nutritional
counseling that amounted to little more than handing out brochures
extolling the virtues of the food pyramid.

One thing is certain: The AAP's recommendation to prescribe cholesterol-lowering drugs to children gives a green light for pediatricians
to scribble millions more prescriptions each year on behalf of the drug
companies. In light of what is readily known about statins, this decision
quite possibly was based on information derived from pharmaceutical
brochures rather than evidence-based medicine.

Statin drugs are so commonly prescribed for adults that most people
assume that the safety of this class of drugs is a well-established no-
brainer. Ironically, it is the measureable loss of brain function that is the
second most common side effect of statins, according to Beatrice
Golomb, M.D., a neurobiologist at the University of California San
Diego. Dr. Golomb has spent years conducting independent research
(read: not funded by Pharma companies) on statin drugs.

"Statins may cause cognitive problems simply because they lower
cholesterol…. Cholesterol is the main organic molecule in the brain
and constitutes over half the dry weight of the brain," said Dr. Golomb
in an interview with *Smart Money Magazine*.

Statin users performed measurably worse on tests of attention and
psychomotor skills in another study that compared before-and-after
performance of patients taking either a statin drug or a placebo for 6

months. The loss may be temporary, according to Matthew Muldoon, M.D., the professor of medicine at the University of Pittsburgh School of Medicine who conducted the study, but it is also possible that statin users suffer longer-term losses in their cognitive abilities.

Parents should be informed at the outset of serious adverse effects associated with cholesterol-lowering drugs, the substantial risks of which are understandably downplayed by drug companies for marketing purposes.

Cholesterol is an important component of the cell membrane of each and every cell in the entire body. Most of the cholesterol inside the human body is made right there, independently of how much cholesterol is eaten in food (cholesterol is found in animal-based foods only). Cholesterol is produced by the body for numerous vital functions, including the production of bile acids that aid digestion of fat and clearance of toxins. Cholesterol is also key in the production of vitamin D for immune system function, calcium metabolism, the production of adrenal hormones that control our ability to handle stress, and the formation of sex hormones.

The drug ads repeat the same message over and over: Statins save lives. But what exactly does this mean? How many lives are saved? "One fewer heart attack per 100 people...to spare one person a heart attack, 100 people had to take Lipitor for more than three years. The other 99 got no measurable benefit," according to *Business Week* in January 2008.

In other words, reported the *British Medical Journal* in May 2006, in order to save one life, 198 people need to take statins for 5 years. According to normal scientific standards, such a pathetically small benefit would be dismissed as statistically insignificant. We must keep in mind, however, that we are talking about medical science here, in which a virtually nonexistent benefit can be heavily marketed to doctors and patients alike and reach the coveted status of being the second most prescribed class of drugs in the world.

The 99 out of 100 people who get zero positive health benefits from their daily dose of statins do at least have something to show: a considerable risk of losing cognitive function, thousands of dollars wasted each year, and daily depleted energy production at the cellular level.

Statin drugs taken as directed deliver a daily dose of a chemical that essentially inhibits the body's innate production of energy. Normal cell function in every single cell throughout the entire body is downgraded each and every day by the ingestion of these drugs. Statins interfere with the body's formation of Coenzyme Q10, essential for the mitochondria in each cell to produce ATP, which is the energy required for carrying out all cellular activities. Proper functioning of all muscle tissue, including the heart—itself a big muscle—is impaired with statin use.

"Statin-induced CoQ10 depletion is well documented in animal and human studies with detrimental cardiac consequences in both animal models and human trials," according to cardiovascular disease specialist Peter Langsjoen, M.D.

"Statins can have significant side effects that have been overlooked or deliberately suppressed. In addition to rhabdomyolysis and liver dysfunction, these include: muscle pain, weakness and fatigue and biopsy evidence of myopathy and tendinopathy…memory loss, global amnesia, difficulty in sleeping and concentration, erectile dysfunction, problems with temperature regulation, difficulty in managing diabetes, and peripheral neuropathy," according to Paul Rosch, M.D., professor of medicine and psychiatry at New York Medical College.

Rhabdomyolysis is a life-threatening, muscle-wasting condition in which the deteriorated muscle tissue enters the bloodstream and overloads the kidneys, leading to kidney failure.

The wild marketing claims that statins are lifesaving drugs are based on a benefit to a very small subpopulation: middle-aged males who have already suffered one heart attack. In this high-risk group only, the use of statins has been shown to reduce the death rate from a second heart attack by about 30 percent. Ironically, it appears that this result is not even related to changes in cholesterol levels but to some other unknown biochemical change caused by the drug.

"For healthy men, for women with or without heart disease and for people over 70, there is little evidence, if any, that taking a statin will make a meaningful difference in how long they live," according to the *New York Times* in January 2008, "Statins have side effects that are underrated…. It's much more frequent and serious than has been reported."

It would appear that the widespread prescribing of statin drugs to people with no preexisting heart disease is yet another Big Pharma victory of public relations and marketing over clinical science. The drug makers have apparently partnered with the AAP so they can now zero in on a huge, untapped market: children.

But does it make any sense whatsoever to place millions of children on a drug that directly inhibits growth and muscle development during the time of greatest growth in their lives, a drug that neither prevents heart attacks nor reduces death except for middle-aged men who have already had a heart attack? And how long will all these children continue taking statin drugs? For the rest of their lives, just as adults do?

It is hardly a secret that the best way to ensure a lifetime of good heart health for children is a healthy lifestyle, including a diet with abundant fresh foods, fruits, and vegetables, free of chemical additives and chemical contaminants, plenty of outdoor activity, high quality rest and sleep, and a loving, nurturing environment.

Do not be surprised if the next time you see your child's pediatrician, he or she tells you that your child has "failed" the cholesterol exam and needs a prescription for cholesterol-lowering drugs. If this happens to you, try asking the good doctor to please explain how a human body in a healthy state could possibly produce a substance within itself that is dangerous to human health.

Breathing Easier Without Asthma Medication

For breath is life, and if you breathe well you will live long on earth.
Sanskrit Proverb

Asthma is a serious breathing disorder caused by immune responses whose timing has gone haywire in the breathing passages. An asthma "attack" is the triggering of three immune responses all at once, initiated by the body in response to a perceived threat—an over-the-top immune response completely out of proportion to the actual threat.

In most cases of asthma, tiny irritants such as dust or pollen particles trigger three immune responses all at once: narrowing of the airways, heavy secretion of sticky mucus, and inflammation in the linings of the bronchial tubes. Other asthma triggers include allergies, medications, exercise, and even certain foods.

The name asthma appropriately comes from the ancient Greek verb *aazein*, meaning shortness of breath or heavy breathing with the mouth open and panting.

According to the U.S. Surgeon General, asthma now affects one in every eight children. Health authorities are at a loss to explain what is causing the asthma epidemic, which seems to primarily be affecting people in modern industrialized societies.

"Despite decades of data, researchers are no closer now to understanding the roots of the asthma epidemic than they were when it first began 20 years ago," reported the Public Health Policy Advisory Board in 2002.

Asthma is the number-one reason children end up in hospital emergency rooms in the United States; as many as 30 million people have asthma symptoms at one time or another in their lifetimes.

Thankfully, death caused by asthma is relatively rare, but it seems that modern medicine has breathed new life into the old saying, "The cure is worse than the disease." Researchers at Cornell and Stanford Universities now tell us that the top-selling asthma medications are responsible for four out of every five deaths from asthma, according to the online *Medical News Today* in June 2006. "We estimate that approximately 4,000 of the 5,000 asthma deaths that occur in the U.S. each year are caused by these long-acting beta-agonists, and we urge that (they) be taken off the market," wrote the researchers.

Now I don't know about you, but I find this news a bit alarming. It makes me wonder what our fearless defenders of public health over at the U.S. Food and Drug Administration (FDA) are doing to protect us. How is it possible that 80 percent of asthma deaths are actually caused by the drugs approved by the FDA to treat the symptoms of asthma? And why is this high percentage of accidental drug-induced deaths insufficient to trigger a drug recall? Shouldn't there at least be one of those little black-box warnings? When and if they finally get around to requiring the black-box warning on the drug's packaging, this message might be appropriate: There is a pretty good chance this drug may kill you, but if it does not, you can breathe a little easier.

In all seriousness, doesn't it appear we could vastly reduce the number of asthma deaths by figuring out alternatives to asthma medication? The apparent logic in the allopathic medical community about asthma is this: Sure, deaths from asthma drugs are a tragedy, but many more people would die of asthma were they not using the drugs. The unspoken assumption is that drugs are the only effective option for treating asthma symptoms, an assumption that appears to be incorrect.

Asthma is commonly referred to as a disease, but I would argue that a more accurate description of asthma is acute dysregulation of multiple immune responses. Each one of the three elements of the asthma "attack" is a normal, life-saving response provided by nature to maintain a healthy immune system—when the timing is correct.

There are times when it is useful and necessary to make the air passages smaller, just as it is sometimes appropriate for the body to produce hefty quantities of mucus to line and protect the airways. There are even times when it is necessary for the immune system to generate a complete inflammatory process to renew the cells lining the breathing passages to restore internal order for healthy breathing.

The name *asthma* describes the condition of all three of these responses being unleashed at the same time. Such a three-part response is major overkill, like attacking the moths in your closet with a 12-gauge shotgun. The shotgun response would obviously be inappropriate, wildly out of proportion to the actual threat posed to your wardrobe, and would likely cause greater damage to your clothes than the moths alone would cause.

"Asthma attacks are increasing even as air pollutants and most other allergens have declined in the U.S. and other developed countries," according to *Reason Magazine* in January 2001. Are asthma sufferers becoming more highly sensitized because fewer environmental irritants are able to trigger more and more asthmatic responses, or is there some other explanation for all the increased hypersensitivity?

"A growing body of research points toward changes in the immune system forced by exposures in the womb or shortly after birth as the cause of heightened sensitivity to allergens, and thus the cause of asthma's rise," reported the Collaborative on Health and the Environment in 2004.

My wife, Nancy, and I found out about sensitization the hard way with our youngest son, Charlie. One night when he was 2 years old, Charlie began having difficulty breathing and started turning a light shade of blue. We jumped in the car and raced down to the emergency room. At the hospital they concluded Charlie was having an asthma attack and gave him asthma medication. We were greatly relieved and grateful when the drugs had an immediate effect. We were given a handful of drug samples to tide us over for a few days until we could get bona fide prescriptions from our family doctor.

"There is no cure for asthma," we were told by the emergency team. "The only thing you can do is treat the symptoms and try to manage the disease."

Thankfully, Charlie never needed to use the asthma drugs after that night because no asthma symptoms ever showed up again. He is now an active 19-year-old who was an energetic soccer player for many years before discovering surfing, which he still pursues with a daily passion. In Charlie's case we discovered right away the sensitizing factor that triggered his breathing distress: cow's milk. Complete avoidance of cow's milk was all it took to "cure" Charlie's asthma at the time.

Researchers are seeking clues in the environment for causes of asthma. Children higher up on the socioeconomic ladder are raised in environments that tend to be incredibly clean, even sterile. One theory is that this ultra-cleanliness can prevent the child's immune system from ever "flexing its muscle" by coming in contact with, and responding to, microorganisms, dust, dirt, and pet dander.

"One of the many explanations for asthma being the most common chronic disease in the developed world is the 'hygiene hypothesis.' This hypothesis suggests that the critical postnatal period of immune response is derailed by the extremely clean household environments often found in the developed world. In other words, the young child's environment can be 'too clean' to pose an effective challenge to a maturing immune system," according to the FDA on its Web site.

Children at the low end of the socioeconomic scale suffer similarly high rates of asthma in this country, but apparently for different reasons than children from more affluent families. For less-advantaged children, the quality of their nutrition is often terribly substandard, and the air quality is poor, with high levels of particulate matter. These kids are also constantly exposed to higher levels of residue from dead insects and the insecticides used to kill them. Kids from both extremes of the spectrum end up with the same result: inappropriately timed immune responses.

Official medical guidelines for asthma focus on the treatment and management of symptoms, but little if any information or guidance is provided concerning the underlying problem of sensitization and how to avoid developing it. Medical remedies seek to suppress the immune responses, whereas more natural, or vitalistic, approaches seek to restore the innate control of immune function and thereby regain appropriate timing of immune responses.

Chiropractic care to restore control of immune responses and reduce or eliminate the need for asthma medication is supported by many anecdotal reports and case studies. It is the apparent ability of the chiropractic adjustment to restore innate signaling throughout the nervous system that accounts for the popularity among parents of this drug-free approach.

To reduce immune sensitization, the first step is to find out which foods and other environmental factors may be the causal factors. Dairy and gluten-containing products top the list of foods linked to hypersensitivity. Not surprisingly, the list of additional items to avoid includes the usual suspects known to interfere with normal healing, such as sugar, highly refined and processed foods, artificial flavors, artificial colors, preservatives, and pesticides, to name a few. It is also helpful to upgrade the diet to include foods containing high levels of noninflammatory nutrients, notably omega-3 fats.

Surprisingly, some standard medical interventions seem to cause immune hypersensitivity in certain children, priming them for asthma attacks. For example, the use of antibiotics in very young children, particularly during the first year of life, leads to a fourfold increased risk of asthma, according to research reported in the journal *New Scientist* in September 2003. A child given a broad-spectrum antibiotic in early life is 8.9 times more likely to suffer from asthma, according to this study.

"The increasing use of antibiotics to treat disease may be responsible for the rising rates of asthma and allergies. By upsetting the body's normal balance of gut microbes, antibiotics may prevent our immune system from distinguishing between harmless chemicals and real attacks," according to the *New Scientist* in May 2004.

Vaccines are also linked to the asthma epidemic. "The odds of having a history of asthma were twice as great among vaccinated subjects than among unvaccinated subjects. The odds of having any allergy-related respiratory symptom in the past 12 months was 63 percent greater among vaccinated subjects than unvaccinated subjects," according to the *Journal of Manipulative and Physiological Therapeutics* in February 2000.

For these reasons, parents may wish to be very conservative in their decision making when it comes to medical interventions for their children, especially since allopathic physicians seem generally unaware of the connection between antibiotics, vaccines, and higher rates of asthma.

In the words of French author Marcel Proust, "Medicine being a compendium of the successive and contradictory mistakes of medical practitioners, when we summon the wisest of them to our aid, the chances are that we may be relying on a scientific truth, the error of which will be recognized in a few years' time."

Perhaps we will all breathe a little easier as more and more parents discover ways to enhance their child's immune development in a natural environment, eliminate common causes of hypersensitization, and thereby completely avoid the frightening and deadly risks associated with common asthma medications.

Sleep Makes the Grade

*That we are not much sicker and much madder than we are is due
exclusively to that most blessed and blessing of all natural graces, sleep.*

Aldous Huxley

The struggle to discover new ways to raise our students' test scores has become a primary focus in schools all across the land. All manner of innovation is being tried to see what works. Special teaching programs with special books, elaborate computer and video instruction, even weekend retreats—we keep scrambling to kick the numbers up just one more notch.

I read in the newspaper the other day of a new pinnacle of dedication to the achievement of higher test scores reached in a nearby school district. Teachers there have begun donating their free time to stay after the bell rings at the end of the day and keep on teaching the kids. For many of the teachers, it just means they are adding additional hours to the extra overtime hours they were already donating to the cause. Of course, teachers are also accustomed to donating their own money to buy classroom materials because the districts do not seem to have much money for such things.

But another trend has surfaced in a few school districts around the country, one that is setting off alarms—or should I say, turning the alarms off. They have found a way to improve test scores, enhance athletic performance, reduce misbehavior and improve attendance. What is happening in these school districts in Virginia, Colorado, Kentucky, Connecticut, and Minnesota that we should know about? Are they trying out powerful new psychoactive drugs? Thankfully, not this time.

A schoolteacher is one who talks in someone else's sleep, according to the old wisdom. Apparently, this is especially true in a typical classroom during the first hours of the morning. "Since the amount of sleep a student gets correlates strongly with academic performance and social behavior, it's important for high schools to have later start times," said William Dement, director of the Sleep Disorders Center at Stanford University.

"Inadequate sleep makes kids more moody, more impulsive, and less able to concentrate. We've known for more than 20 years that sleep deprivation makes it difficult to learn," said pediatrician Alan Greene, M.D. He believes chronic poor sleep results in daytime tiredness, difficulties with focused attention, difficulty controlling behavior and a lower threshold for irritability and frustration.

Sounds to me like a list of symptoms for Attention Deficit Hyperactivity Disorder (ADHD). In fact, a list that was nearly identical to the list above appeared in a recent magazine advertisement for antidepressants. "Yes or no: do you have trouble with grades, school or work, an inability to concentrate, troubled relationships with family and friends, and loss of control over behavior? If you said yes to all of these, the problem may be depression. The good news—you can get treatment and feel better!" I'm thinking a recommendation for more sleep is not what the drug company had in mind.

I wonder how many kids in our town are downing daily doses of powerful stimulants to treat what is actually sleep deprivation? Especially since a common trait among children diagnosed with ADHD is restless, interrupted sleep. Then, to make matters worse, we put stimulant drugs into these children's nervous systems, which is known to degrade the quality of their sleep even more. But finding natural ways to help kids sleep better seems to improve their behavior, even if lack of restful sleep is not the core problem.

If you've ever had teenagers, you are no doubt familiar with conversations that go something like this: "You've got to go to bed right now."

"Why?"

"Because you have to get up early and go to school."

"But I'm not sleepy!"

"Well, go to bed anyway."

"Why should I go to bed if I'm not sleepy?"

"Because you need the sleep!" And so on.

Parents may feel that teenage defiance and procrastination are the causes of late-night texting or talking on the telephone, chatting on Internet chat rooms, watching TV, and basically doing everything else besides going to sleep. But Brown University Professor Mary Carskadon tells us these are not acts of rebellion. Researchers have "measured the presence of the sleep-promoting hormone melatonin in teenagers' saliva at different times of the day. They learned that the melatonin levels rise later at night than they do in children and adults—and remain at a higher level later in the morning."

That explains why rousting our slumbering sons and daughters out of the sack in the morning is like trying to raise the dead. If people were meant to pop out of bed, we'd all sleep in toasters, goes the old saying.

Professor Carskadon claims that it is time for American schools to face the biological facts. "Children learn from kindergarten on about the food pyramid....But no one is teaching them the life pyramid that has sleep at the base." In her view, efforts to improve student achievement should begin with starting school later in the morning.

It appears we need to adapt to the idea that adolescents have different sleep patterns than adults, alert in the evening and bleary-eyed in the morning. Doctors pretty much agree that children and teenagers need nine and a half hours of sleep or more every night. How many hours are your teens getting? I'm pretty sure mine do not get enough sleep during the school year.

There are more than 13,000 school systems in the United States. Estimates are that the vast majority of high schools across the country still start at about 7 a.m. "There is no magic number about when to start school, but closer to 8 is better than closer to 7, and closer to 8:30 is probably better than 7:30," according to Professor Carskadon.

Of course, changing the hour that school starts is not a simple matter and costs money. Some communities have considered a start-time change only to later abandon the effort when community opposition prevented it. Concern centers on lost time for after-school activities and athletic practice and difficulty for students to keep after-school jobs.

Making a time change obviously affects everyone, including siblings, parents, teachers, administrators, district personnel, and the rest of the community. But an organization called Start Later for Excellence in Education Proposal (SLEEP) reports that many of those fears may be unfounded.

"While any change requires adjustments, experience in other jurisdictions indicates no major problems. A year after the Minneapolis high schools switched to an 8:40 a.m. start time, 92 percent of parents reported being happy with the change."

According to SLEEP, schools "have found that participation in sports and other extracurricular activities actually improved after going to later start and end times....Coaches in Wilton [Connecticut] noted that the year after the bell schedule change was one of their best athletic seasons, with the high school winning several state athletic championships."

All this talk about sleep really got me wondering though, what about the rest of us? Our whole country is 24-hourized, sleep-deprived, over-stimulated, and just plain tired.

We must not forget history's lesson that sleep deprivation has played a pivotal role in some of the worst catastrophes in modern history. For example, the nuclear accident at Three Mile Island happened in the wee morning hours, reportedly caused by drowsy workers with poor judgment. The gas leak in Bohpal, India, in 1984 was blamed on inattentive, fatigued workers. The explosion of the space shuttle Challenger has been blamed on decisions made by managers who hadn't slept much for days. The Chernobyl nuclear meltdown was linked to sleepiness of the workers there. And who can forget the Exxon Valdez that went aground in Alaska? Faulty orders from a sleep-deprived first mate are blamed for that one.

Sleep is not an option, it is a necessity. The only issues regarding sleep are the quality and the quantity of the sleep we get. Research suggests that more sleep could be a key to higher academic achievement. Do you suppose getting more sleep could change the health and safety of the entire world?

"Sleep is the golden chain that ties health and our bodies together," said Thomas Dekker. He may be right. I'm not sure though, I need to sleep on it.

Getting Over Cold Medicine

*A family is a unit composed not only of children but of men, women,
an occasional animal, and the common cold.*

Ogden Nash

"**V**ery young children commonly come down with common
colds." Agreement with this statement is universal among
parents, pediatricians, drugmakers, and even the Food and Drug
Administration (FDA). However, as to the question of whether or not
over-the-counter (OTC) cold medicine is helpful to little ones suffering from a cold, there is far less agreement.

"It's important to point out that these medicines are safe and effec-
tive when used as directed," said Linda A. Suydam, president of the
Consumer Healthcare Products Association, quoted in *The Washington
Post* in October 2007.

"Clearly, the products don't work and are unsafe," said Joshua M. Sharfstein, M.D., Baltimore Health Commissioner, quoted in the same *Post* article.

Could these two views be any further apart? Hardly. Can cold medicines be safe and effective while at the same time be unsafe and not work? No. Which means one of these people is making up a fantasy version of the truth, commonly known as "lying." Who do you suppose is making things up, the spokesperson for the cold medicine industry or the doctor from the Baltimore Health Commission?

When it came to getting a cold in my family, we accepted the traditional wisdom about colds: Take a cold remedy and get over it in seven days, take nothing at all and you will have that cold for a week.

The American Academy of Pediatrics (AAP), surprisingly, seems to agree with the traditional view on this particular subject and recommends against medicating young children to treat cold symptoms. Drugmakers, on the other hand, have been spending about 50 million bucks each year to convince parents to buy OTC drugs to treat cold symptoms. Cold medicine advertising seems to work just fine, because sales reportedly jumped 20 percent last year and were expected to climb again this year—that is, up until last week.

That is when fourteen cold medication formulas for infants were pulled from store shelves across the country, just seven days before an FDA committee was slated to begin investigating the drugs.

"An FDA review prepared for next week's meeting describes dozens of cases of convulsions, heart problems, trouble breathing, neurological complications and other reactions, including at least 54 deaths involving decongestants and 69 deaths involving antihistamines," reported *The Washington Post*. It is estimated that there are 500 deaths per year associated with children's cough and cold medicine, according to the journal *Pediatrics* in December 2008.

Dr. Sharfstein long ago alerted the FDA to widespread problems with the drugs after a total of 900 Maryland children under age four suffered an overdose in a single year, 2004.

"Given that there are serious consequences, including death, associated with the use of these products without compelling reason to use them, why are they being marketed for children?" Sharfstein asked. "The contrast between the state of the evidence and the displays in drugstores could not be more stark."

"There is no evidence that the products are effective for young children, and there is evidence they can be unsafe, even at the usual doses. This is not just about misuse," he said, noting that the dosages typically used are untested estimates based on studies in adults. "That's why we are asking the FDA to clearly label these products against use by children under age 6," according to *The Washington Post*.

It is an interesting paradox that doctors are in the position of pleading with the agency in charge of drug safety to try and halt the medical treatment of nonmedical symptoms of a self-limiting health challenge. The preferred recommendations sound familiar: bed rest, lots of fluids, chicken soup if you like, and large doses of vitamin C.

"Whatever grandma recommends that's nutritious, get the kid to eat it...It's better than all the over-the-counter stuff," said Daniel Rauch, M.D., director of the pediatric program at NYU Medical Center, quoted in the *New York Daily News* in October 2007.

"These medications were never designed to cure colds but only to treat cold symptoms," said Katherine Tom-Revzon, pediatric pharmacist at the Children's Hospital at Montefiore in the Bronx. "In children under 2, there was little evidence they were effective, anyway," reported the *Daily News*.

A robust, innate immune response in both children and adults requires the *expression* of symptoms, not the *suppression* of symptoms. The symptoms of a cold are self-limiting and benign for the vast majority of well-nourished people and serve to activate and bolster immunity. Infections with colds viruses are part of a lifelong process of encountering microbes in the environment and mounting an innately directed, short-term inflammatory response that results in permanent cellular memory and strengthened immunity.

"This is not a situation in which pediatric data are lacking and we are unable to say one way or the other," wrote Jay Berkelhamer, M.D. in a letter to the FDA. Dr. Berkelhamer is the national president of the American Academy of Pediatrics. In multiple studies, they have "been found not to be effective in this population at all," according to Berkelhamer, quoted in an Associated Press article in October 2007.

The FDA ignored its own advisory committee's advice to require labels that caution against use of the drugs in children under 6 years old. The agency instead stood by as the drug makers voluntarily changed their labeling to caution against using the drug in children under 4 years old. But how effective are words of caution on the packaging—packaging that winds up in the trash anyway the moment the parent arrives home with the medicine?

If the FDA really wants to save lives and prevent overdose with unnecessary medications, new and innovative measures are needed. Why not require the drug companies to chip in a week or two of profits from sales of the drugs each year to fund an "unsales campaign" using clever "nondrug" television ads that recommend you *not* ask your doctor? Consumers could greatly benefit from learning that colds are not a medical problem. Parents of the world need to know that drugs intended to suppress cold symptoms also depress natural immunity and cause disruption of healthy cellular function.

New "Please Don't Drug Me" ads could let the public in on a secret many health professionals already know: The body is fully capable of healing itself from colds and just about everything else. Parents should be encouraged to throw away all the antihistamines, decongestants, and fever-lowering drugs, and then feed their child a bowl of hearty soup before tucking them back in bed.

Placebos, Real Drug Problems, and a Real Solution

It requires a great deal of faith for a man to be cured by his own placebos.

John L. McClenahan

The placebo is perhaps the most fascinating and mysterious entity in the history of medicine. The humble placebo has been hailed as the safest, most effective medicine ever discovered, with some even claiming that the history of effective medical treatment itself is a history of the placebo response.

Placebo is Latin for "I shall please."

The placebo response has been observed for centuries, not only with the classic inert, or "sugar," pills, but also with other faked medical protocols such as sham surgeries and simulated medical procedures. The placebo response mechanism is not well understood, but the patient's belief that the sugar pill or sham surgery is going to help appears to trigger an authentic, inborn healing response.

Allen Roses, M.D., an executive vice president for a preposterously enormous pharmaceutical company, in public remarks made a couple of years ago, outlined our real drug problem, paraphrased here: Prescription drugs do not work most of the time.

But before we delve into the basis for his comments, ask yourself this: What do you think is the biggest drug problem facing our country? Illicit drug abuse? That is a big problem for sure, especially for the poor drug dealers out on the streets. Think of the unfair competition they suffer from doctors who can scribble prescriptions 24/7 all year long with no worry of being arrested for pushing wildly powerful and addictive mind-altering and painkilling drugs. In point of fact, illicit drug abuse does not even come close to the problems we are having with prescription drug abuse. These days, far more emergency room visits and deaths result from overdosing on legal drugs than on the illegal ones.

What about antibiotic overuse and abuse? Dr. Richard Besser of the Centers for Disease Control (CDC) has admitted that there are tens of millions of unnecessary and inappropriate antibiotic prescriptions written each year in this country alone, and the problem keeps getting worse. So bad, in fact, that some medical researchers predict we are at the brink of catastrophic outbreaks of infectious disease caused by killer microbes with resistance to every antibiotic we have.

Perhaps you are concerned about the epidemic of prescribing powerful mind-altering drugs in all age groups from toddlers to the very elderly for newly named psychiatric disorders. Antipsychotic drugs are now the most widely prescribed class of prescription drugs, yet we have no clear understanding of how or why these drugs work. Not to mention that we have no idea what will happen in the course of the lives of the thousands of two-year-olds who are now strung out on prescription narcotic stimulants intended to modify their beahvior.

Maybe you were thinking that the astronomical cost to taxpayers for Medicare drugs is our biggest problem. If so, that just proves you are not a shareholder in the Big Pharma drug cartel. Just ask anyone who owns drug company stock and they will tell you that the current Medicare system works just fine. Bilking the government for billions of dollars each year is still as easy as pie; it turns out that the roadblocks against fraud legislated by Congress are pretty much constructed of smoke and mirrors only.

What about unintentional death caused by prescription drugs and medical errors? Researcher Gary Null, Ph.D., in his report *Death By Medicine*, calculated a total of 999,936 annual deaths resulting from medical interventions that started off with good intentions but then went south. This last point is a tragedy of unimaginable proportions, but it is seldom spoken of in polite conversation and rarely debated in the mainstream media.

Finally, this is Dr. Roses' description of what he believes is the true and fundamental problem with prescription drugs: "The vast majority of drugs—more than 90 per cent—only work in 30 or 50 percent of the people. I wouldn't say that most drugs don't work. I would say that most drugs work in 30 to 50 percent of people."

What? Just think of it, one-half to two-thirds of all people who take prescription drugs receive no benefit from the drug whatsoever. No benefit at all, but still they get the substantial risks of debilitating and life-threatening adverse reactions. Within the Pharma industry, this is not news at all, but discussing this fact within earshot of the public was apparently a serious breach of etiquette for a drug company executive. Industry secrets such as this are intended to remain locked in those basements several stories underground in the same location Big Pharma keeps all those other millions of industry skeletons.

Colleagues of Dr. Roses in the pharmaceutical world were distressed and annoyed by his comments, to put it mildly. Public relations departments had to shift into code-red-priority, emergency damage control to hastily clarify what the good doctor actually meant to say, which apparently was: "Take your pills because drugs are good for you and make you healthy! Ask your doctor."

The admission by Dr. Roses that most people gain no benefit from prescription drugs was remarkable not only for its frankness, but also because it affirmed that active drugs work no better than placebos where it counts the most: in the real world.

The artificial laboratory conditions imposed by drug trials in no way resemble reality, because only healthy people are used in the testing, people are given only one drug at a time, and the tests last for a few days or at most a couple of weeks. Meanwhile, out in the real world, sick people are taking three, four, five, or a dozen other drugs every single day, medications recommended to be taken for a lifetime, not just a week or two.

To put into perspective a meager 30 to 50 percent effectiveness for FDA-approved pharmaceuticals, let us compare this to the track record of the lowly placebo. Fifty years of research has documented patient benefit from using placebos 30 to 70 percent of the time. A recent study suggests that even when the doctor tells the patient right up front they are being given a placebo—a completely fake drug with no possible benefit—a measureable and pronounced benefit still occurs. An important point to remember here is that the placebo response is in no way inferior to whatever beneficial response may be triggered by active drugs, yet placebos avoid side effects. No side effects that is, unless the placebos are doctored with chemicals to mimic the side effects of the drug being tested, reportedly a common practice these days.

So how bad is America's drug problem? Prescription drugs and medical errors accidentally kill about 616 people every single day, or about 225,000 people a year, according to Barbara Starfield, M.D., M.P.H., in the *Journal of the American Medical Association* July 2000. As Moliere correctly noted, "Most men die of their remedies, not of their illnesses."

The federal government, to its credit, sometimes actually steps forward to try and defend American citizens from harm caused by already-approved prescription drugs. What this means is that FDA commissioners occasionally hold hearings and then demand that a black-box warning be printed on the drug package to warn doctors just how dangerous the drug is. I wonder when our regulatory geniuses will realize how ineffective this "strongest possible precaution" is, considering that the good doctor writing the scrip never gets to see the actual drug packaging?

As an example of the complete ineffectiveness of federal government protections for the American public, let's take antibiotics. I don't mean you should actually take an antibiotic, we should just look at what we know about them. For more than 20 years, various government agencies have repeatedly sent out strongly worded press releases and verbal warnings to doctors insisting that they quit writing millions of worthless antibiotic prescriptions for conditions that antibiotics cannot possibly affect. The result? Abuse and overuse of antibiotics continues to be a thriving business. And the superbugs in American hospitals could not be happier.

Occasionally, the government asks us for help in its thankless task of reducing the unintended collateral damage caused by well-intentioned interventions prescribed by overworked medical professionals. For example (I am not making this up), if you find yourself in the hospital, Uncle Sam asks that you do your part to reduce human-to-human microbe transmission. Your job is to ask each doctor if he or she washed his or her hands before coming into your room. As you can imagine, complying with this request may trigger an adverse reaction, because some doctors just seem to get snippy when asked when they last washed their hands. But do not be intimidated, just remind the doctor that you are under strict orders from the United States Government to ask these questions.

Here is another tip to help avoid the kind of tragic and irreversible mistakes in the operating room that have become urban legends, such as removing the wrong kidney, amputating the wrong foot, or removing the wrong breast. On the day of surgery, borrow the nurse's indelible felt tip marker and write instructions on yourself to remind the doctor where to operate. Apparently, surgeons usually recall the "why" of the operation, but an alarming number of them get confused about the "where." Mark the correct spot on your body with "Operate Here." Then, on the opposite side write "Do Not Operate Here." It is hoped that this tip will help your surgery start off on the right foot. Or was it the left foot? Regardless, it is best to write the instructions on yourself before you have been given anesthesia.

As for the massive problem of unintentional prescription drug death and disability, I am pleased to announce that a remedy is within our grasp. A course of action everyone can live with has finally been worked out—by yours truly. This remedy has the potential to save the suffering of millions of people while allowing the drug companies to continue reaping billions of dollars in obscene profits. Meanwhile, doctors will just continue writing loads of prescriptions and still receive all the free pens, coffee mugs, calendars, meals, generous speaking honoraria, and getaway trips to the Bahamas that they are accustomed to receiving.

Let us do the math. Real drugs work 30 to 50 percent of the time, and placebos work 30 to 70 percent of the time, which gives placebos a slight edge. Drug companies can just start mixing them willy-nilly inside the little pill bottles. The pills will look the same and smell the same. Nobody will know whether they are taking a real pill or a placebo. The outcomes will be approximately the same, except there will be fewer dead patients and other nasty side effects.

Clever workers at the drug-manufacturing plants will no doubt eventually figure out how much cheaper it would be to just fill all the bottles 100 percent with sugar pills and leave out the dangerous drugs. Decades of clinical science tells us that it will not even matter when the active drugs go completely missing.

And so my fellow Americans, let us embrace the available science in favor of prescription placebos. Let us look forward to the day when the worst adverse reaction to prescribed drugs will be dental problems caused by eating too many placebos.

One Flu Over the Cuckoo's Nest, or Dead Chickens Never Lie

If medical statistics were compiled by statisticians who had no interest in the outcome, the drug industry would topple into the dust.

Robert Catalano

Author's note: This story begins a few years ago when public health officials were freaking out about the avian flu.

Lying on the plate in front of me was a savory, cooked-to-perfection, dead chicken. As the delicious aroma rose into my nostrils, I was blinded by a flash of insight, a realization that might effectively eradicate the terrifying avian flu "not-a-question-of-if-but-when" pandemic. The constant crowing on the news about the devastating possibility of a full-blown pandemic was still scaring the pants off citizens all over the world. If you could believe the pundits and pandemic experts, the sky was falling. Were they just being chicken, or were they reanimating the fable of Chicken Little?

I lifted my fork for another bite of the perfectly roasted, tasty fowl. Delicious. My wife, who is vegetarian, politely averted her eyes and lightly dabbed the corners of her mouth with a napkin while I chewed slowly, savoring each succulent morsel. I wondered how it was possible that dead chickens could taste so good while simultaneously threatening to bring down the entire civilized world.

Here, for the record, is the insight that momentarily blinded me: Public health leaders the world over need to stop counting their dead chickens before they hatch. That's right, those leaders need to stop counting dead chickens before they hatch another plan to vaccinate every human with experimental vaccines and questionable drugs.

Just to get an idea of how bad the avian flu thing really was up to that point, I consulted the news headlines. Sure enough, it appeared that the worst fears of the fearful and the scariest predictions of the prediction makers were coming true: Dead chickens had just been discovered on the other side of the world in Upper Faraway, a remote village in the diminutive republic of Eastern Highlandia.

The venerable scientists who made this alarming discovery had been dispatched by the World Health Organization (WHO) to find out how many dead chickens might be lurking in the tiny mountain community. The scientists were a small part of the army of WHO researchers fanning out across the planet to count dead chickens to help world health leaders understand the spread of the terrifying avian flu.

Curious villagers lined the streets to give a hearty welcome to the three half-frozen men who survived the 300-mile vertical climb riding on the backs of yaks. The last time the village had received visitors from the outside was six years earlier in 1999, when computer technicians made the perilous journey.

The purpose of the earlier trip was to prepare the village for the impending and certain-to-be-hideous Y2K disaster. (Remember Y2K, the predicted disaster that failed to crash even a single computer?) "But this time," the WHO scientists urgently proclaimed to the villagers, "there is an impending bird flu disaster that is absolutely, positively 100 percent guaranteed to be monstrously hideous!" With earnest faces the scientists tried to explain that the only question remaining about the looming avian flu pandemic was how soon it would arrive.

Unable to speak the natives' language, the scientists took off their heavy arctic gloves and used improvised hand gestures to try and communicate with the villagers. At some point about an hour into their hand signals and gyrations, they were led to the town's shack where all the dead chickens were stored. The scientists cautiously stepped inside and discovered that several chickens were indeed hanging upside down on wooden pegs in neat rows.

The scientists attempted to act out the strange behaviors that an avian flu–stricken, dying chicken might exhibit before toppling over dead, and in response the villagers began clapping their hands and joined in dancing the funky chicken with the learned travelers. Someone broke out some warm mead and soon the big party was moved inside the town hall for feasting, heavy drinking, and dancing that lasted all through the night. In the inevitable morning-after hangover of foggy confusion, none of the scientists could recall where they left their Official Avian Flu Dead Chicken Test Kit.

Nevertheless, in the official report submitted to the WHO by the scientists, it was confirmed that several dead chickens had indeed been discovered, and all were, in fact, deceased. The cause of death was listed as "unknown," although foul play was suspected by one of the scientists who wrote in his notes, "It looked as though someone had wrung the neck of every last one." Unsteadily, the three scientists mounted their sturdy yaks and headed back down the treacherous mountainside, but only after each villager had given them a good-bye hug.

Back in the modern world, preparations for the big and scary pandemic continued apace. The instant collapse of the poultry industry was predicted to occur as soon as the first dead American chicken was discovered to have the flu. The loss of confidence in the safety of eating poultry was already well underway in France and a few other countries. People apparently didn't believe the experts who told them there was no way to get bird flu from eating cooked dead birds, so the entire bird industry was expected to be brought to its knees in a matter of days.

The prepandemic hysteria created some of its own serious side effects, including overcrowded emergency rooms, hospitals, and airports; schools and businesses were closed, and forced quarantine plans were at the ready, plus a whole raft of red-alert military-style contingency plans for responding to civil disobedience that might ensue.

Meanwhile, government officials in the United States quietly sifted through the proposed federal budget to locate a few billion more taxpayer dollars to send over to the poor, cash-strapped pharmaceutical companies to pay for millions of doses of experimental vaccines. Of course, they were using the avian flu strain in their new vaccine that could not possibly end up being the one that might actually cause a pandemic, because no mutation had occurred yet. But this was business as usual, a clever application of the classic strategy, "Don't worry about trying to make scientific sense as long as you can make loads of dollars."

If only we could inoculate our public health leaders with common sense. Independent scientists have repeatedly shown that our health leaders' enthusiasm for annual flu shots is not supported in the medical literature. The abysmal track record of flu shots suggests that pandemic flu shots will prove to be equally ineffective.

Our government also got busy stockpiling warehouses full of Tamiflu, the drug called "useless" by the Vietnamese doctor who actually tried it out on real avian flu patients. It is reported that using the drug actually makes the virus more resistant. Good job, team! In response, company spokespeople assured the public that the drug really is effective, pointing to the strong numbers they came up with in their laboratory studies.

As a side note, the solution to this drug resistance conundrum is so obvious, how did the pharmaceutical boys miss it? We should simply send everyone who contracts avian flu to the laboratory where Tamiflu was tested, since that is the only location where it seems to work fighting the symptoms of the virus.

Now, fast-forward several years past the pathetic showing of the avian flu, and the dreaded swine flu was charging onto center stage. Once again the public health alarms were sounded, only this time the WHO got so excited about the pig virus going viral that they changed the definition of pandemic and immediately pegged the risk of swine flu sweeping the globe as the highest-possible threat. Ever.

In hindsight we can see how the story unfolded. Not only did the swine flu fizzle, but that year the flu season around the globe was less eventful and even more mundane than usual. The specially prepared, government-funded, scantily tested pork shot was pitched and promoted more heavily than all the top-selling car brands in the world combined, but less than a third of the population could be goaded into getting jabbed.

Seriously folks, has any flu pandemic in the last 70 years caused even a fraction of the annual deaths and disability for adults caused by heart disease, cancer, stroke, diabetes, and even death from properly prescribed drugs? No. Are children much sicker today than they were a generation ago, and are they the first generation with a predicted lifespan shorter than their parents? Yes. Does any of this have to do with infectious disease? No.

Is it possible that our public health leaders' focus on imaginary flu pandemics and the promotion of vaccines and drugs as the only possible solution to such perceived catastrophes is based on nothing more than the unassailable political and economic power of Big Pharma and their quest for profitability?

Public health authorities have yet to learn the vital importance of honoring nature, nurture, and nutrition, the time-tested and truly effective ways to build up the health of individuals and our entire population. How can we convince our health leaders that creating good health is the very best way to prepare our immune systems for any possible exposure to whatever viruses and other microbial challenges may arise?

The real reason we found bird flu in flocks all over the globe for the first time ever was because laboratories around the world were massively testing for it for the first time ever. The only threat from the swine flu was a perceived possibility that it would somehow mutate and gain the ability to spread from human to human.

It is becoming apparent to more and more people that the efforts of our global health leaders to fight infectious influenza would serve humankind better if the focus were shifted to improved nutrition and sanitation for the world's population.

The time has come for health authorities to stop counting dead chickens before they hatch and to stop nitpicking sick piggies in the poke. The scientifically misguided and wasteful preparations being made for World War Flu should henceforth be laid aside and replaced with something scientifically guaranteed to help everyone be healthier, such as supplementing the world's population with vitamin D3.

FDA-Approved Viruses in our Victuals

*If people let the government decide what foods they eat and what
medicines they take, their bodies will soon be in as sorry a state
as the souls who live under tyranny.*

Benjamin Franklin

I was sitting in my folding plastic chair the other day, inside my new
ten-by-ten plastic antiseptic isolation tent in the living room (available online for about 3,000 bucks, plus shipping and handling). The
electric air sanitizer was busily humming away, and, as far as I could tell,
I had done all I could to separate myself from the jillions of invisible
germs all around me, especially the SARS germs, avian flu germs, and
now the swine flu germs the government and all the news broadcasters
were talking about. One week earlier, just to be safe, I gave away my pet
chicken named Little (a certifiable avian), and my potbelly pig named
Porkchop (a swine if there ever was one).

I was deep in a debate with myself about the risk of exposing myself to hordes of invisible microbes by climbing out of my tent, versus the benefit of venturing out to a medical clinic for a mumps booster shot, a flu shot, a swine flu shot, and shots for meningitis, hepatitis, tetanus, chicken pox, shingles, pneumonia, polio, hangnail, and whatever else they had. Paranoid? Not me, just trying to do as I'm told by our public-health specialists.

Just then I glimpsed a curious newspaper headline out of the corner of my eye about viruses and government health authorities. With growing alarm, I read the accompanying article and realized that the turkey, pickle, and cheese sandwich I had just eaten might have been teeming with government-approved viruses. What in the world?

The government has apparently decided that adding viruses to food is a good thing, because a virus cocktail has been approved by the Food and Drug Administration (FDA) to be sprayed on prepared, ready-to-eat meat and poultry. How gross is that? For years we have all been taught to be terrified of viruses, and now we are supposed to chow down on them?

"This new virus spray approved by the hot dogs up at the FDA for processed meats is pure baloney," observed one FDA critic.

Indeed, when I read that the FDA, the federal agency in charge of the safety of our food supply, had suddenly endorsed the spread of viruses on food, it left me very confused. That is, until I learned the reason for the spray: to try and clean up processed meat products that are contaminated with one particular bacterium, listeria.

The new virus spray for processed meat is only the latest FDA-approved method for battling bacteria. This new strategy joins food irradiation (the zapping of our food with ionizing radiation) to sterilize the food surface and feeding antibiotics by the barrel to animals just to keep them alive on corporate farms under horrifyingly unhealthy conditions. I wonder, would any of these remedial steps even be necessary if Big Food was forced to clean up its act instead?

"Listeria is a reasonably nasty bacteria found in soil, water and the intestines of food-producing animals. Animals who carry listeria can spread it to meat, dairy products or to other products that roll around a processing plant en route to your plate," reported ABC News.

The FDA historically has done all it could to help the food industry make more money, whether it is approving untested genetically modified crops or covering up contamination problems in the food factories, so I guess I should not be too surprised.

This new virus spray is a mixture of six viruses known as "phages," or bacteria eaters. Reportedly this is the first time an infectious microbe has been approved for use in a food fight to kill a competing infectious microbe growing on the food.

Keep in mind that the residue that remains on the meat following the battle to the death between viruses and bacteria must inevitably end up in the digestive tracts of those who eat it. The FDA tells us this is not a problem, at least not a direct problem, because the viruses do not attack human cells. But what about the billions upon trillions of friendly bacteria present in the digestive system, the gut flora that must remain healthy so that we ourselves may remain healthy? Will the viruses bring their war against bacteria to our friendly bacteria by mistake? It sounds as if friendly fire could be a big problem in this new war.

Not to worry, says the FDA, these viral armies have been "trained" to attack only listeria. Just imagine those boot-camp training sessions: All right, you maggoty viruses, listen up. As soon as you soldiers pass through the mouth and head down that tube for the stomach, you will immediately stand down, permanently. And that's an order!

It appears that we have no choice but to trust the FDA's word on the sensibility of this whole virus project. But has the FDA overlooked the fact that the listeria bacteria are not going to lay down and give up without a fight? Microbes have notorious skills for quickly evolving resistance to whatever is eating them. What happens then? Will the FDA order a troop surge and begin deploying more viral battalions with stronger, more highly trained viral troops? How do you train a virus, anyway? And what else do they put in the spray, preservatives and weird, toxic chemicals and heavy metals like the ones used in vaccines?

And here's another thing, the toxins produced and excreted on and in the meat by the bacteria before they are killed by the victorious virus armies will not be eliminated or altered in the least, no matter how high the casualty rates go for the bruised and beaten bacteria.

Perhaps the greatest threat of this new viral war on bacteria is the vast number of unpredictable immune responses in human beings when millions of people are eating bacteria-killing viruses day after day, year after year. Phages are foreign proteins, and foreign proteins have been known to directly provoke a range of immune responses in susceptible individuals. Is it possible our already over-the-top, raging epidemics of asthma, allergies and autoimmune disorders could get even worse as a result of virus-infected victuals?

I can only imagine that many more viral sprays will be needed to kill all the other types of bacteria lying in wait on our contaminated cold cuts. I am told that a new army of spray-on viruses is being trained to fight salmonella, while another viral squad of assassins with E. coli in its crosshairs is not far behind.

People at risk of listeria infection include pregnant women, elderly folks with compromised immune systems, and the very young. You might think that the FDA's job would be to first warn these at-risk groups to avoid eating processed meat until the contamination problems can be resolved and then go about forcing corporations to clean up their facilities and change their meat-processing methods. Instead, the FDA has given industrial food producers the green light to continue producing filthy food while launching a vast experiment, the exposure of millions of Americans to "safe and edible" viruses.

The combined number of deaths caused by infection from all three bacteria, listeria, salmonella, and E. coli, together is less than 600 per year, according to the Centers for Disease Control, and the National Vital Statistics Report. Has the FDA not noticed that more than 100,000 persons die each year from properly prescribed, FDA-approved drugs? That works out to about 600 deaths every couple of days. Statistics suggest that citizens have more to fear from FDA-approved medicines than we do from bacteria on our baloney.

As for me, I'm transformed. I've become "pro-biotic." After making peace with my trillions of personal, resident microbes, I decided to stop worrying about the wild viruses and bacteria. But you can be sure I'm going to avoid contact with combat-trained, FDA-approved viruses if at all possible. I'm converting my isolation tent into an aboveground swimming pool, my pet chicken Little is back, and so is Porkchop. The next time I order a sandwich, I'm telling them to hold the mayo, hold the mustard, and hold the virus. In fact, please just give me a tomato and cucumber sandwich.

Drug Advertising Works

Advertising may be described as the science of arresting the human intelligence long enough to get money from it.

Stephen Leacock

"Doc, I'm pretty sure I need some of those green pills—you know, like the ones on television."

"Really? What are your symptoms?"

"Well, I feel like I'm the guy in the TV commercial standing next to the telephone. I can't pick it up because I'm scared to death who might be calling me."

"Ah, sounds to me like a classic case of Electronic Communication Initiation Rejection Disorder (ECIRD). You need the little yellow pill."

"Wait a minute, doc, the little yellow pill is just for women. I saw that commercial just the other day."

"No Jimmy, I'm afraid you're wrong. The woman in that commercial suffers from Social Avoidance Dysfunctional Anxiety Disorder (SADAD). She needs the orange pill with black polka dots, remember?"

"Oh."

"Don't worry, Jimmy, I'm a doctor. Not knowing what color pill you need is a common mistake. Drug ads, I mean Pharmaceutical Educational Public Service Announcements, can be confusing. Remember the one with the panicked mother standing outside the kindergarten classroom? She has Primary Retrograde Personality Deficit Complex (PRPDC). She needs that little yellow pill, and so do you."

"Are you sure, Doc? What would the guys think if they knew I was taking a girly pill?"

"Jimmy, you need to just trust me here, because I'm a real doctor. Listen," he said, lowering his voice, "If you were any other patient I probably wouldn't tell you this, but the little yellow pill, the orange pill with black polka dots and the green pill are really all the same drug, just packaged and marketed differently."

"You're kidding."

"No, that's the honest truth. The drug salesman was here just yesterday and told me the secret. I do get a bigger kickback, I mean inducement reward, for prescribing the yellow one, but since you like the green one, no problem."

The story you have just read may be true, but I doubt it. I made it up. The names have been changed to protect the...uh, well, actually I changed the names to protect myself from lawsuits brought by Big Pharma for making fun of how the drug lords push legal drugs: on television, on the radio, in magazines and newspapers—not to mention all the advertising on the Internet.

In the old days, the snake oil salesmen would pull up their horse-drawn wagons on the edge of town, pull in a crowd, and proceed to dazzle the audience with a song and dance about how great their remedies were. Now they just pull into your living room and deliver their hokum through the TV screen. At least these days there aren't horses leaving road apples scattered around on the living room carpet when they hitch up and leave.

Ever since 1997, when it became legal to advertise on radio and TV, the public airwaves have become more and more saturated with direct-to-consumer (DTC) drug advertising. This has literally changed the way people go about getting their prescription drugs. We now self-medicate with the newest, least-tested, most expensive, most heavily advertised prescription drugs out there. No longer do we need to limit our self-medicating habits to a six-pack of beer, a few shots of scotch, or some other recreational drug.

"A bartender is just a pharmacist with a limited inventory," according to folklore. Just step into the office of your choice, tell the doctor which color pill you want based on which advertisement you like best, and, bingo! Four minutes (or maybe four hours) later you walk out of the doctor's office and head to the pharmacy clutching in your hot little fist the prescription you asked for.

Doctors really do write the exact prescription people request about 70 percent of the time, according to Ray Strand in his book, *Death by Prescription*. Drug companies are well aware of this fact. That is why they do not even blink about spending $4 billion every year on DTC marketing.

Only the United States and New Zealand, among all countries in the world, allow DTC drug advertising. The absurd claim that these ads are somehow educational or provide important patient information would be laughable if the consequences weren't so tragic.

The normal ups and downs of daily life are steadily being transformed by advertising into made-up diseases. We learn that these new, invented diseases must be treated with powerful, dangerous and expensive drugs. In the process, we are diverted from traditional healing wisdom and robbed of natural solutions for creating health, navigating the challenges of life with a clear head, and dying peacefully with dignity.

Deliberate and systematic destruction of common sense in primary health care is a side effect of DTC drug advertising. A noble goal would be an outright ban on prescription drug advertising over the public airwaves.

What about regulating the ads instead of instituting a total ban? Any attempt at regulating the DTC beast other than a total ban must fail. As noted by Solon, one of the seven wise men of ancient Greece, "Laws are like spider's webs which, if anything small falls into them they ensnare it, but large things break through and escape." We know regulation would fail because the FDA already fails miserably at regulating the content of advertising that goes out to doctors in drug company brochures and medical journals. Unfortunately, doctors routinely decide which drugs to prescribe based on these marketing materials.

This in itself wouldn't be so bad if only the claims in these brochures and journal ads came from verifiable scientific evidence and data. Alas, it is simply ad copy written by professional marketers whose only goal is to sell drugs. "Only 6 percent of the brochures contained statements that were scientifically supported by identifiable literature," according to the *British Medical Journal* in February 2004.

"We chat together; he gives me prescriptions; I never follow them, so I get well," wrote the French playwright, Molière.

Perhaps we should all follow his example. When the man on the TV says to ask your doctor if the pink tablet is right for you, consider just saying no to drugs. Remember, "Every great advance in natural knowledge has involved the absolute rejection of authority," said Thomas Huxley. The time has come to revoke Big Pharma's permission to come into America's living rooms and hawk their dangerous wares.

Jimmy's story has a happy ending. While he was still in the doctor's office, Jimmy suddenly got clarity and came to a decision. "Doc, I just changed my mind. You are the one who needs help, you are suffering from Chronic Pharmaceutical Psychobabble Hyperdementia Disorder (CPPHD). You can keep your big green pills, little yellow pills, the orange ones with black polka dots, and all the rest. But please don't flush that toxic pharmaceutical crap down the toilet, you'll end up poisoning everyone downstream."

Asleep at the Wheel

Sleep 'til you're hungry, eat 'til you're sleepy.
Author Unknown

Insomnia has recently been elevated by the drug industry to the status of a dangerous menace to public health. Sleep deprivation is now being blamed for depression, auto accidents, and high disease rates. In the old days things such as worry, poor diet, too much coffee, and late-night partying were considered to be the cause of insomnia, but that was before drug company executives woke up and smelled the coffee. That is when the campaign against wakeful nights began in earnest; the time had come to help people understand that a lack of pharmaceuticals circulating in the blood causes lost sleep.

Drug company scientists were tasked with transforming insomnia from a relatively modest problem into a massively serious disorder affecting pretty much the whole nation. Insomnia needed a new reputation as a

medical condition so serious it required daily doses of heavily advertised medication for a lifetime. Spin doctors had their work cut out for
them if they were to convince people that it was worth the risk of suffering some unique and troubling adverse reactions in order to gain a
little bit of sleep.

These researchers rolled up their sleeves and got to work, sparing no
expense. Years of effort and hundreds of millions of dollars were spent
creating mountains of data, cobbling together complex computer models of sleep, analyzing sleepy people, and crunching lots of big numbers
in order to better understand and do battle with insomnia, the mysterious disorder of the darkness.

At lengthy conferences attended by hundreds of doctors, the results
of rigorous testing of numerous chemical compounds on rats, dogs,
monkeys, and computers were pored over and discussed. Finally, after
creating just the right chemical concoction and choosing the correct
pill name, shape, and color by polling thousands of people in hundreds
of focus groups, it was time. The results were reported in corporate
boardrooms with impressive four-color bar graphs, pie charts, and
emotion-laden videos. It was time to sound the alarm; time to broadcast
a wakeup call to the whole nation: ask your doctor which sleeping pill
is right for you.

Cha-ching! Pharma's massive marketing arm sprang into action and
launched a multimillion-dollar, multipronged promotional blizzard
accompanied by fabulous media fanfare and fake news segments on the
evening news. Doctors foolish enough to persist in prescribing an old-
fashioned glass of warm milk, a shot of whiskey, or counting sheep for
insomniac patients found themselves warned, scorned, and publically
humiliated for straying from the flock. Only a quack would deny that
the era of better living through chemicals requires prescribing only the
latest patented drugs. Strong nations require really strong bedtime
medication—it only makes sense.

For those who remain unconvinced that insomnia is a serious medical problem, I offer the following self-evident proof: several new
brands of sleeping pills have been approved in the last couple of years.
And if the chief of the U.S. Food and Drug Administration (FDA) gets
his way, the superhighway of fast-track approval will soon be paved with
gold to facilitate the rapid delivery of truckloads of new, improved,
extra-strength pills to pharmacy shelves all over the country faster than
you can say, "Honey, please stop reading and turn out the light."

"Fast-track" approval is a drug industry term that translates as, oh
sure, we promise to someday maybe get around to testing those pills,

but first we'd like to start selling them and bank several billion bucks. As you can imagine, the fast-track shortcut is very popular with the drug industry. Massive marketing campaigns for new drugs seem to generate much higher sales when drug companies do not have to try and explain weird and debilitating side effects that are detected during the actual drug safety trials they promise to do later at some unspecified future time.

As a side note, keep in mind that the term "side effect" has one meaning for medical consumers and a much different one for drug industry insiders. In standard English, a drug with side effects is a drug that may seriously and permanently screw up your health and possibly kill you. For Pharma companies the terms side effect and adverse reaction mean annoying little public relations problems. No matter how serious the adverse event, details can be obfuscated with scientific-sounding bull and extra advertising. It is simply a cost of doing business these days.

Consider, for example, antidepressants. Presumably, depressed people who seek professional help from a psychiatrist do so in hopes of finding a happy solution. But not long after antidepressants were approved, marketed, and widely prescribed, doctors began noticing a common, pervasive, and troubling side effect: antidepressants make many people feel like killing themselves. The compassionate response from the drug companies was immediate: "Golly. Bummer! But hey, listen, the FDA has already approved our pills, so go complain to someone who might give a rat's whisker about your problems."

A major pharmaceutical CEO complained recently that the media is forcing the FDA to focus too much on unwanted side effects of new drugs and not enough on the benefits. Perhaps he makes a good point. How many people would willingly subject themselves to say, having botulism injected into their face to get rid of a few wrinkles if they understood that sudden death is a potential, and very real, side effect? That is exactly why side effects are listed on the backside of magazine ads in print so tiny they are illegible, and spoken in the background in television ads so rapidly the words only vaguely resemble English.

Which brings us back to sleeping pills. Consider the recent mean-spirited display of news reporting when a few minor side effects showed up for people taking their prescribed sleeping aids. Sleepwalking is listed as a side effect, and this is nothing new of course, but it does become dangerous when the drugged sleeper walks out of his or her home and onto a busy intersection or else deftly climbs out an upper-story window and discovers, quite by accident, a startling new adverse event called sleep-falling.

Another rather interesting and distinctive new side effect is called sleep-eating. It seems that the newer sleeping pills cause some people to climb out of their beds, walk into the kitchen, and ravage the contents of their refrigerator, ripping open packages of food and indiscriminately scarfing down every morsel in sight. One report described a woman who realized she had a drug-induced sleep-eating disorder only after a mysterious weight gain of 100 pounds, even though the average person might reasonably be expected to become suspicious after gaining 30 or 40 pounds. You might have thought that finding empty ice cream cartons under the blankets and food wrappers scattered over the kitchen floor every morning would have raised red flags earlier too. This woman's huge problem brings new meaning to the term heavy sleeper.

But the absolutely most truly exciting new side effect of these pills is sleep-driving. You may recall that sleeping aids were originally advertised as beneficial for reducing auto accidents. As it turns out, though, people arrested for impaired driving increasingly test positive for sleep medication in their bloodstream instead of alcohol. Anecdotal stories are accumulating of people who wake up behind the wheel of their car as it crashes into another car or suddenly open their eyes to find themselves motoring down an unknown road in an unknown part of town at 3:00 a.m. with several cupcake wrappers and an empty bag of pork rinds on the seat beside them.

Maybe the drug company CEO makes a good point in his complaint. Maybe we should view these bizarre new side effects of sleeping aids as benefits instead of problems. Imagine how much time we could save if we could keep sleeping right through our morning shower and breakfast and then not even wake up until we had driven all the way to work. Could sleeping aids be one of those long-promised wonder drugs that will change everyone's life for the better? Just think, if everyone of us could begin sleeping through our daily activities all day long, the bedrooms in our houses could be converted into something more useful. Imagine having plenty of room in the house to stack case upon case of potato chips, saltines, chocolate chip cookies, candy bars, and tiny donuts, not to mention strategically placing refrigerators around the house with ample capacity to satisfy the midnight-munching needs of an entire household of sleep-eaters.

If the drug companies work this idea properly, sleepwalking could give way to sleep-working. Come to think of it, though, promoting drug-induced sleep-working may not work because this is an art form already practiced successfully by millions of people in cubicles all over America who require no sleeping aids to nod out all day long. In all fairness, credit for this concept must belong to Heraclitus, who commented way back in 500 BC, "Even sleepers are workers and collaborators in what goes on in the universe."

Ultimately, Big Pharma's profit analysts may scrap this particular off-label marketing scheme for sleeping aids for a different reason: if people could sleep the day away on the job, fewer of them would feel depressed. Obviously, that would cut into the billions of dollars in profit from the sale of antidepressants to all the millions of people currently numbing their brains against the daily drudgery of work and, worse, the dread of impending unemployment. In the end, the poor pharmaceutical makers may realize it is best after all to market their sleeping aids to a much smaller audience: people who actually suffer from intractable insomnia.

But wait, says sleep researcher Jim Horne, Ph.D., sugar pills work just about as well as sleeping pills for insomniacs, and you don't have to worry about being pulled over by a cop and arrested in your pajamas. "They can help to a limited extent, but people generally don't realize just how little extra sleep they actually give you," said Horne.

The National Institutes of Health looked into that question and found that real sleeping pills make people fall asleep only 12.8 minutes faster, and add only 11 minutes more to a night's sleep than do the fake pills. Not only that, said Horne, sleeping aids "should only be taken as a short-term emergency or maybe longer if you are very ill and in pain."

His caution echoes statements from the Medicines and Healthcare products Regulatory Agency in the U.K. That agency warns that sleeping pills are a short-term treatment only, to be used only by people who are acutely distressed. Specifically, the agency warns of psychiatric adverse effects such as nightmares and hallucination. The most common side effects from frequent use include dizziness, headaches, facial swelling, allergies, and addiction.

"If your insomnia goes on for more than a week or so, it is usually your waking life that is the problem," according to Professor Horne. "The number one reason people have difficulty falling asleep or keep waking up is that they are stressed or anxious. If that's happening you need help organizing your life and learning to relax," he said.

When it comes to sleep, the bottom line was perhaps best summarized by playwright Wilson Mizener, "The amount of sleep required by the average person is five minutes more."

The War on Breast Cancer

War is the unfolding of miscalculations.
Barbara Tuchman

In 1971 President Richard Nixon committed our nation to the war on cancer. This seemed the right thing to do because at that time an American woman's chance that she would have breast cancer in her lifetime was 1 in 20. Tragically, by 2005 the lifetime risk was reportedly almost three times as great, 1 in 7.

This trend may sound to you as if the war on cancer has not been going too well so far. Obviously, you are not one of the experts at the National Cancer Institute (NCI), because if you were, you would say we are winning the war on cancer. I am not making this up.

"In war," said Ramman Kenoun, "there are no winners." It would appear that in the war on cancer there are no mathematicians either.

Breast cancer is deadly, killing ever-greater numbers of women in the United States and other industrialized countries every year. Breast cancer tops the list of cancer deaths among women in this country, annually claiming the lives of more than 40,000 women.

The incidence of all types of cancer has climbed to such epidemic proportions during recent decades that a man living in the United States now has a nearly fifty-fifty chance he will have cancer during his lifetime; for a woman, the chance is greater than 1 in 3, according to the journal *Oncologist* January 2007. Within a single generation we have seen an increase in cancer of approximately 56 percent for men and 22 percent for women. An estimated total of 569,490 cancer deaths occurred in the United States in 2010, according to the American Cancer Society (ACS).

So how can the NCI tell us we are winning the war against cancer when the evidence tells us that virtually every type of cancer is clobbering us worse than ever? Apparently all it takes is the wave of a statistical magic wand over the numbers. You'd be surprised how much this dresses things up for the cameras and enhances fundraising.

To be fair, the mortality rate for men with lung cancer has dipped slightly because fewer men now smoke, but the apparent reduction in overall mortality rates cited by the cancer industry is a statistical sleight of hand that reflects earlier detection rates, not increased survival from improved cancer treatments, according to John Bailar, M.D., former editor of the *Journal of the National Cancer Institute.*

"The five year cancer survival statistics of the American Cancer Society are very misleading. They now count things that are not cancer, and, because we are able to diagnose at an earlier stage of the disease, patients falsely appear to live longer. Our whole cancer research in the past 20 years has been a failure. More people over 30 are dying from cancer than ever before.... More women with mild or benign diseases are being included in statistics and reported as being 'cured.' When government officials point to survival figures and say they are winning the war against cancer they are using those survival rates improperly," wrote Bailar in the *New England Journal of Medicine* September/October 1990.

Official statistics include easily curable cancers, nonspreading cancers, melanomas, and precancers that are not cancer at all, according to Tanya Harter Pierce in her book *Outsmart Your Cancer*. She cites the example of ductal carcinoma in situ (DCIS), which reportedly has a cure rate of 99 percent. Since this accounts for 30 percent of all breast cancer types, inclusion of DCIS numbers is misleading because it skews the survival statistics and cure rates of breast cancer favorably upward by 30 percent.

Once we remove the rose-colored glasses proffered by the NCI and the American Cancer Society, we can see we are losing the great war on cancer quite miserably. Perhaps, as Jeanette Rankin has suggested, "You can no more win a war than you can win an earthquake."

"Find the Cure" is the rallying cry of pink-themed events around the country, designed to raise awareness and to raise money. These activities are linked to well-funded national media campaigns to promote the search for elusive pharmaceutical-based cures for cancer.

Could it be that the focus on finding "the cure" is holding us back from real progress in saving lives by looking at environmental causes and how women may protect themselves from environmental exposures? Only an estimated 5 to 10 percent of breast cancer has a genetic base, according to the National Institutes of Health on its Web site, and yet the billions of dollars spent on research continues to be funneled into finding the gene that "causes" breast cancer.

The primary sponsor and mastermind of the annual Breast Cancer Awareness month and corporate pink-washing is AstraZeneca Pharmaceuticals, maker of the controversial drug widely prescribed for breast cancer, Tamoxifen. All media campaigns for the cure on television, radio, and in print must be approved by AstraZeneca. Interestingly, Tamoxifen is a substance known to cause cancer, according to the National Institute for Environmental Health Sciences, reported by the *New York Times* on May 16, 2000. Even more ironic is the fact that AstraZeneca also manufactures Acetochlor, an organochlorine pesticide suspected to be a causal factor of breast cancer.

It seems entirely possible that the reason we have not shifted to a strategy of prevention from the expensive and ineffectual search for pharmacological cures is blatant conflict of interest. "Breast cancer is simply not a preventable disease," says the NCI, whereas the ACS has stated, "there are no practical ways to prevent breast cancer—only early detection." It must take many tons of sand to enable so many researchers to keep their heads buried when it comes to the relationship between breast cancer and the environment. Perhaps the sand is trucked in free of charge by the pharmaceutical/chemical-producing companies for just this purpose.

"For years the ACS demonstrated its allegiance to the multibillion-dollar cancer drug industry by aggressively attacking potential competitors through its Committee on Unproven Methods of Cancer

Management, created to 'review' unorthodox or alternative therapies. This committee, staffed by 'volunteer health care professionals,' invariably promoted mainstream, expensive, and arguably toxic drugs patented by major pharmaceutical companies and opposed alternative, or 'unproven,' therapies, which are generally cheap, non-patentable, and minimally toxic," according to Samuel Epstein, M.D., University of Illinois professor, in *Tikkun Magazine* November/December 2000.

But the evidence is in: It's the environment, stupid! Researchers examined the results of 21 different studies and published a report called *State of the Evidence 2004: What Is the Connection Between the Environment and Breast Cancer?* The research was sponsored by two non-profit groups not funded with Big Pharma money, the Breast Cancer Fund and Breast Cancer Action.

"This new report offers the clearest evidence yet that the rise in breast cancer incidence is linked to exposure to radiation and toxic chemicals. Medical x rays, pesticides, household cleaning products, personal care products and some pharmaceuticals—these are just a few of the multiple and chronic exposures contributing to this epidemic," said Nancy Evans, a health science consultant with the Breast Cancer Fund.

Other known risk factors include use of oral contraceptives, more than four years of hormone replacement therapy, alcohol consumption, bovine growth hormone in milk (rBGH), exposure to secondhand cigarette smoke, chlorinated chemicals, paint and varnish dyes, household cleaning products, and personal care products, according to the Breast Cancer Fund.

The institutionalized war on breast cancer has evolved into a big business with budgets in the billions. "When you add it all up, Americans have spent, through taxes, donations, and private R&D, close to $200 billion, in inflation-adjusted dollars, since 1971," according to the *CNN Money* Web site in March 2004.

Meanwhile, our sworn enemy in this war is still pummeling us and gaining ground. Worse, casualties include alarmingly high death rates caused by the friendly fire of toxic pharmacological agents, as well as the collateral damage caused by toxic screening methods using ionizing radiation.

Traditionally, mammography has been the frontline strategy for early detection of breast cancer. Ironically, these x rays are not only surprisingly unreliable for early detection, they are an additional risk factor for breast cancer. A standard four-film mammography study exposes a woman to a dose of ionizing radiation sufficient to increase her risk of breast cancer 1 percent every single time, according to Dr. Epstein. Ten years of showing up to get painfully squished for the recommended annual mammogram yields a 10 percent increased risk for breast cancer.

"Mammograms increase the risk for developing breast cancer and raise the risk of spreading or metastasizing an existing growth," warns Dr. Charles B. Simone, a former clinical associate in immunology and pharmacology at the NCI.

A controversial change to guidelines for mammography screening was proposed in November 2009 by the U.S. Preventive Services Task Force, a federal advisory board. The group concluded that mammography is not very effective in screening for cancer detection in younger women, whose breasts tend to be denser. The group also said that yearly mammograms should not be automatic at age 40, and for women ages 50 to 74, routine mammography screenings should be done only every 2 years. These new and moderately restrictive guidelines, based on researching years of clinical outcomes, were met with strong opposition from the mammography industry.

"The mammography industry conducts research for the [American Cancer] Society and its grantees, serves on its advisory boards, and donates considerable funds. DuPont, a major manufacturer of mammography equipment (in addition to being a major petrochemical manufacturer), is a primary supporter of the ACS Breast Health Awareness Program. The company sponsors television shows and other media productions touting mammography; produces advertising, promotional, and informational literature for hospitals, clinics, medical organizations, and doctors; produces educational films; and lobbies Congress for legislation promoting access to mammography services. In virtually all important actions, the ACS aligns itself with the mammography industry, failing to pursue viable alternatives to mammography," according to Epstein.

What other options are there? Thermal imaging is a remarkable, noninvasive technology truly capable of early detection. Tragically, this underutilized technology is dismissed and even maligned by many cancer experts. Thermal scans can detect a neoplasm in its earliest stages of development, when the tumor consists of as few as 256 cells. Compare this to mammography, which cannot detect a tumor until it has been developing for 8 years and grown to a size greater than 4 billion cells!

But the very most important detection method of all is the breast self-exam a woman should be practicing regularly. According to Dr. Epstein, the ACS admits that "at least 90 percent of the women who develop breast carcinomas discover the tumors themselves."

The war on cancer has primarily involved cutting, poisoning, and burning out the symptoms of cancer in millions of people, leaving the underlying causes intact, while disputing the significance of environmental factors for developing breast cancer. Natural and inherently safe methods of cancer prevention and treatment have been consistently marginalized, persecuted, and even criminalized by the efforts of the cancer establishment. This has perpetuated ignorance among mainstream medical practitioners about the crucial role of diet, supplemental nutrition, and lifestyle factors that can prevent and promote healing from cancer.

Each year more corporations join in the phony pink parades with endless fundraising promotions to funnel more money into Big Pharma companies to find the cure. Some of these corporations are the very ones whose manufacturing processes and products spread pollutants through the environment and into our bodies, increasing the risk of all sorts of cancer.

Each year more women are conscripted to walk, run, ride, swim, roller skate, and even turn cartwheels for the cure, but all the corporate pink-washing and awareness events fall far short of making actual progress toward greater breast health for women. The time has come for healing. We need to create the political will that is necessary to eliminate sources of toxicity in the food supply, in the environment, and, yes, even in mainstream medical care—starting with toxic cancer screening and treatments.

The Institutes of Medicine (IOM) in December 2011 recommended a list of actions on its Web site that a woman may take to reduce her environmental risk of breast cancer: "The IOM concludes that women may have some opportunities to reduce their risk of breast cancer through personal actions, such as avoiding unnecessary medical radiation throughout life, avoiding use of estrogen–progestin hormone therapy, avoiding smoking, limiting alcohol consumption, increasing physical activity, and, for postmenopausal breast cancer, minimizing weight gain."

The time has come to declare that the war on breast cancer has been a tragic and counterproductive diversion from the real task of helping woman experience greater breast health naturally. We need the biggest education campaign ever to help every woman understand the environmental risk factors for breast cancer, how they may be avoided, and the positive steps that are available and known to promote breast health and overall health.

Fluoridation Nation

Any man can make mistakes, but only an idiot persists in his error.

Cicero

"Water, gentlemen, is the one substance from which the earth can conceal nothing. It sucks out its innermost secrets and brings them to our very lips," wrote Jean Giraudoux. It turns out that water also sucks out the dirtiest of industrial secrets, which the public is then compelled to swallow without asking questions.

By coincidence, Giraudoux's words about water were written in 1945, the same year fluoridated water was first brought to American lips through the municipal water supply of Grand Rapids, Michigan. And so began the Great War on Cavities.

Water supplies in the cities of America on that day became a Weapon of Mass Medication. The great cavity war was framed as an incredible modern public health advance, the use of new technology to enhance children's dental health. Unfortunately, as Mr. Giraudoux also later observed, "Everyone, when there's war in the air, learns to live in a new element: falsehood."

The so-called father of fluoridation, Trendley Dean, D.D.S., began his assurances in the 1930s that the addition of fluoride to water was "safe and effective," even "necessary" for strong bones and teeth. Dr. Dean many years later reportedly gave courtroom testimony on two separate occasions that his original claims were incorrect, because they were based on invalid statistical information. Unfortunately, his retractions came too late to derail or even slow the fluoridation train.

A law was passed in 1995 in California requiring fluoridation of all municipal water systems. Too bad for the citizens of the city of San Diego and other locales in the state where voters have repeatedly voiced opposition to water fluoridation at the ballot box. In compliance with state law, fluoride began to flow through the tap into millions of California households during the following decade. Let us acknowledge this mandate for what it is: Fluoridation Without Representation.

What exactly does water fluoridation of municipal water supplies mean, anyway? Does it mean we add the molecule calcium fluoride, which is naturally present in water to a varying degree already? No. Do we add pharmaceutical grade sodium fluoride such as the stuff your dentist applies to the surfaces of your teeth (and pharmacists once sold as cockroach poison)? Nope, not that either.

The answer is in a riddle: What hazardous industrial waste product is extremely dangerous to handle, toxic to all living things, and very expensive to dispose of unless you happen to sell it as a medicinal product to be dumped in municipal water? You guessed it, we are talking about a solution of hydrofluorosilicic acid, the noxious waste that is scraped out of industrial smokestacks. Pretty amazing, isn't it? And here's a bit of irony: We are paying money to Chinese industries to export their hazardous waste to us so we can dump it into American municipal water systems.

What do you suppose are the other tasty ingredients in the fluoridation solution? "The fluorosilicic acid is also contaminated with small traces of arsenic, cadmium, mercury, lead, sulfates, iron and phosphorous, not to mention radionuclides," according the *Earth Island Journal*.

"In promoting the use of the pollution concentrate as a fluoridation agent, the ADA (American Dental Association), Federal agencies and manufacturers failed to mention that it was radioactive. Whenever uranium is found in nature as a component of a mineral, a host of other radionuclides are always found in the mineral in various stages of decay. Uranium and all its decay-rate products are found in phosphate rock, fluorosilicic acid and phosphate fertilizer," according to investigative journalist George C. Glasser.

The scientific and ethical arguments against fluoridation are so significant that one must ask: How is it possible that fluoridation laws are enacted against popular will? Perhaps, as Upton Sinclair remarked, "It is difficult to get a man to understand something when his salary depends on not understanding it." We need to follow the money trail in order to understand why politicians and bureaucrats enable fluoridation to keep coming back like a bad penny.

No self-respecting money trail would be caught dead without a few bodies of evidence buried in the ditch alongside, a smoldering scandal or two lying across the path, and shredded bits of inconvenient science littering the trail—and the fluoridation trail is no exception. It leads right to the doorstep of fertilizer and aluminum producers, who—instead of paying thousands of dollars per ton to clean up their toxic waste—have transformed their enormous hazardous-waste disposal liability into a multimillion-dollar profit stream. "According to recent estimates, the phosphate industry sells approximately 200,000 tons of silicofluorides (hydrofluorosilicic acid and sodium silicofluoride) to U.S. communities each year for use as a water fluoridation agent," according to the *Quarterly Journal of the International Society for Fluoride Research*.

Americans already ingest significant amounts of fluoride in beverages and processed foods. We know this because a minimum of 32 percent of American children and adolescents already display physical signs of fluoride poisoning called fluorosis, the discoloration and pitting of the teeth, according to the Centers for Disease Control (CDC) survey published in August 2005. This news was announced with the standard bland assurances that fluorosis is a "strictly cosmetic" problem.

Really? Since when is lower intelligence a strictly cosmetic problem? "The development of intelligence appeared to be adversely affected by fluoride in the areas with a medium or severe prevalence of fluorosis....A high fluoride intake was associated with a lower intelligence," according to a study in the journal *Fluoride* in November 1995. Fluoride was included on a list of "emerging toxic substances" in *The Lancet* in November 2006, because it is increasingly linked to lower IQs in children and brain damage in animals.

"In Canada, we are now spending more money treating dental fluorosis than we do treating cavities. That includes my own practice," according to Hardy Limeback, Ph.D., D.D.S., former President of the Canadian Association of Dental Research. Canada is among the handful of countries in the world that fluoridates some of its public water supplies.

"I believe that fluorine does, in a mild way, retard caries, but I also believe that the damage it does is far greater than any good it may appear to accomplish. It even makes the teeth so brittle and crumbly they can be treated only with difficulty, if at all," according to George W. Heard, D.D.S.

This whole fluoridation thing started out with a promise of preventing cavities. How's that going so far? The largest dental health survey ever done in the United States was carried out by the National Institute of Dental Research and published in the *Journal of Dental Research* in February 1990. More than 39,000 children in 84 different communities were examined, and the number of decayed, missing, and filled tooth surfaces was compared among children living in fluoridated versus non-fluoridated communities. The data showed that the fluoridated water saved less than 1 percent of children's tooth surfaces from decay. That is approximately one surface of the 128 tooth surfaces in a child's mouth. The benefit of ingested fluoride for dental health turns out to be virtually nonexistent.

And what of the toxicity? For some reason, when the fluoridation floodgates were opened up in California, the information pipeline was shut down completely. Where were the warnings for the many people who need to completely avoid fluoride exposure to preserve their health? Babies up to 1 year old, pregnant moms, the elderly, and anyone with kidney problems, thyroid problems, liver problems, diabetes mellitus, or cardiovascular problems need to be as fluoride free as possible. The last thing these people need is to drink fluoridated water.

The U.S. Department of Health and Human Services (DHHS) has prepared a list of those people at high risk for fluoride toxicity. Following are excerpts from the *Agency for Toxic Substances and Disease Registry* in April 1993:

"Existing data indicate that subsets of the population may be unusually susceptible to the toxic effects of fluoride and its compounds. These populations include the elderly, people with deficiencies of calcium, magnesium, and/or vitamin C, and people with cardiovascular and kidney problems. Because fluoride is excreted through the kidney, people with renal insufficiency would have impaired renal clearance of fluoride....Impaired renal clearance of fluoride has also been found in people with diabetes mellitus and cardiac insufficiency....People over the age of 50 often have decreased renal fluoride clearance....Postmenopausal women and elderly men in fluoridated communities may also be at increased risk of fractures." From that brief list, it would appear that the majority of Americans are "unusually susceptible" to the toxicity of fluoride.

Fluoride is classified scientifically as "very toxic." And just how toxic is that? More toxic than lead and almost as toxic as arsenic. The toxicity rating of lead is between 3 (moderately toxic) and 4 (very toxic). Arsenic is rated slightly above 4, whereas fluoride rates precisely a very toxic 4, according to *Clinical Toxicology of Commercial Products, 1984.*

Even healthy kidneys are able to clear less than 50 percent of the fluoride taken into the body, so fluoride accumulates in the bones and stays there for life. The ingestion of fluoride permanently deposits a substance more deadly than lead right next to the blood cell factories of the body, in the bone marrow.

If you are one of the millions on the list of Americans for whom even the tiniest exposure of fluoride is a bad idea, you need fluoride-free water. Removing fluoride from tap water at home is not simple, requiring the purchase of equipment to either distill the tap water or filter it using reverse osmosis. Eating organic foods and juices is another way to reduce exposure to fluoride.

Perhaps our regional health leaders are reluctant or even embarrassed to post warnings about the known safety problems caused by the addition of hydrofluorosilicic acid to the public water supply. Then again, maybe they are unable to say anything because doing so would jeopardize their jobs. For whatever reason the information is not forthcoming, much of what we do know about fluoride is highly disturbing.

Fluoride is an endocrine disruptor that was used for decades in Europe as a drug to depress thyroid function to treat overactive thyroid. Alarmingly, the dosage once prescribed to reduce thyroid activity is about the same amount ingested by people in many U.S. communities today.

The biological effect of fluoride on living cells is the disruption of enzyme activity, which accounts for its capacity to disable dental bacteria that create dental caries, or cavities. Unfortunately, the ingestion of fluoride also disrupts the enzyme activity that maintains life in human cells.

In October 2006 the Food and Drug Administration (FDA) stated that makers of fluoridated water could no longer claim it reduces the risk of dental cavities in infants. The American Dental Association announced only 1 month later that babies up to 1 year old should avoid fluoridated water altogether because they are at high risk of developing dental fluorosis.

Evidence now links fluoridation to an increased risk of cancer. Researchers reported finding "an association between fluoride exposure in drinking water during childhood and the incidence of osteosarcoma among males," in a study from the Harvard School of Dental Medicine in May 2006. The authors noted that there was a fivefold increased risk of bone cancer for boys exposed to fluoride levels commonly found in American water supplies.

An increase in lead levels in children's blood caused by drinking fluoridated water is also linked to serious societal problems. "At the environmental level, our research has found that environmental factors associated with toxicity are correlated with higher rates of anti-social behavior....Communities using silicofluorides also report higher rates of learning disabilities, ADHD, violent crime, and criminals who were using cocaine at the time of arrest," according to a Dartmouth University study published in September 1999.

Other research indicates that long term exposure to fluoridated water weakens human bone. "The prevalence of hip fractures was highest in the group with the highest water fluoride," reported the *Journal of Bone and Mineral Research* in May 2001.

"A review of recent scientific literature reveals a consistent pattern of evidence—hip fractures, skeletal fluorosis, the effect of fluoride on bone structure, fluoride levels in bones and osteosarcomas...[fluoridation] proponents must come to grips with a serious ethical question: is it right to put fluoride in drinking water and to mislead the community that fluoride must be ingested, when any small benefit is due to the topical action of fluoride on teeth," stated the *Australian and New Zealand Journal of Public Health* in 1997.

Fluoridation enthusiasts assure the public that the level of fluoride added to municipal water is "optimal" and "safe," but providing the rate of fluoridation in a given water supply is meaningless. What matters is the actual amount an individual ingests. Obviously, people who drink lots of tap water will ingest far more fluoride than those who drink only small amounts of water.

The U.S. Public Health Service reported in 1991 that people living in cities with "optimal" water fluoridation may easily receive a total daily fluoride exposure exceeding 6.5 milligrams per person per day. That amount is more than 600 percent above the officially recommended "optimal" amount.

Water is just the first item on the list of substances that expose us to fluoride. We ingest fluoride from toothpaste, mouthwash, dental treatments, soft drinks, juice, commercially raised fruits and vegetables (grown with fluorine-containing pesticides, herbicides and fertilizers), processed and canned food, wine, beer, coffee, and tea, not to mention the ever-increasing amount of fluorine pollution in the environment.

A common belief holds that decision making in modern times no longer relies on superstition and politics, but is based on modern scientific reasoning. If that is true, why do so many modern skyscrapers have no thirteenth floor, and why do we add toxic industrial waste to our drinking water? According to Andrew Mathis, "It is bad luck to be superstitious."

The myth that fluoride is an essential nutrient required by the human body for proper bone and tooth health was long ago laid to rest scientifically. Those preaching the fluoride gospel today are either badly misinformed, under the influence of powerful economic interests, or both.

Historically, the rate of cavities in developed countries around the world has trended downward uniformly, regardless of whether or not the water was artificially fluoridated. The credit for improved dental health around the world belongs to improved nutrition and better dental hygiene.

"In summary we hold that fluoridation is an unreasonable risk. That is, the toxicity of fluoride is great and purported benefits associated with it are so small—if there are any at all—that requiring every man, woman and child in America to ingest it borders on criminal behavior on the part of governments," said J. William Hirzy, Ph.D., research scientist with the Environmental Protection Agency.

Government databases are overflowing with empirical evidence confirming that water fluoridation is a seriously bad idea. I look forward to the day when our profluoridation health leaders will think with their brains (before the fluoride destroys their cognitive function), examine the evidence for themselves, and change their minds about water fluoridation. Many have already done so. Hardy Limeback is a prominent Canadian dentist and longtime leader in his profession who completely reversed his position on fluoridation. He explained in an interview that dentists "have absolutely no training in toxicity. Your well-intentioned dentist is simply following 50 years of misinformation from public health [authorities] and the dental association. Me, too. Unfortunately, we were wrong."

In community after community, when the facts about fluoridation are presented to the citizenry and a vote is taken, fluoride gets flushed. In the first half of 2011 alone, eight communities in the United States voted to end fluoridation of their municipal water.

Ultimately, as Robert Dickson, M.D., pointed out, "Dental decay is a condition associated with poor nutrition, overuse of sugary foods and drinks, poor dental hygiene and lack of good quality, basic dental care."

The time has come for American and Chinese industries to find some other way of disposing of hydrofluorosilicic acid besides forcing it down the throats of the American public while pretending that it protects the health of anything other than corporate bottom lines.

Killer Vitamins

A child of five could understand this. Fetch me a child of five!
Groucho Marx

A curious front-page story had me scratching my head earlier this week. It concerned the intrepid scientists at the National Institutes of Health (NIH) who claim to have carefully studied the question of daily multiple vitamin/mineral use and found the evidence supporting this practice to be "especially thin."

This surprising revelation by an "independent panel of experts" suggested to me one or more of the following possibilities.

The good doctors on the panel either (1) misunderstood the question; (2) limited their search for evidence to prehistoric cave art in France; or (3) were acting out revenge against their mommies for forcing them to take vitamins as children.

There is a fourth possibility that came to mind: Perhaps the NIH panel members are secretly working to help the drug companies who want to take over the $23-billion-a-year vitamin supplement industry.

The leader of the august panel at the NIH, Dr. J. Michael McGinnis, in a moment of startling candor admitted, "We don't know a great deal."

If only they had just switched off the microphones right then and there, ended the press conference, and gone home. Instead, McGinnis went on to say, "We're concerned that some people may be getting too much of certain nutrients."

This observation, while certainly true, struck me as considerably less than profound. To be fair, his comment did at least demonstrate a vague awareness among panel members that epidemic levels of heart disease, stroke, type II diabetes and cancer are somehow related to people eating too much of the wrong nutrients.

However, when I think of people overdoing the wrong nutrients, I tend to picture very large people wolfing down triple-patty-one-pound cheeseburgers with bacon and sausage and a side of cheese fries, rather than someone throwing back a handful of vitamins with a glass of water.

The NIH attack follows at least two other major hit pieces against vitamins recently. In previous months, both *The Wall Street Journal* and ABC Nightly News lambasted vitamins for being unproven for their effectiveness, virtually unregulated and worrisome because they may actually cause harm.

I have to admit I was shocked to hear that vitamins are dangerous and may actually cause harm. Just to be safe, I left my vitamins lying on the kitchen counter while I did a little investigating.

I could not help wondering though: Is it possible the NIH panel members had confused vitamin pills with prescription pills? Perhaps the gentlemen had wandered into the wrong conference room, mistaking a debate on the dangers of prescription drugs for the debate on vitamins. Talk about dangerous: More than 2,000 people die every single week from pharmaceutical drugs—and that's counting only the ones that are properly prescribed and properly ingested at the prescribed doses and time intervals.

Just to find out for myself the level of danger posed by my vitamin pills, I went to the bookcase and pulled out my *Junior Detective Deadly Pills Forensics Manual*. The bold-faced directions on page 1 told me everything I needed to know, "Count the dead bodies. Dangerous pills always leave dead bodies lying around."

Obviously, it was time to check with the proper authorities to find out just how many dead bodies have been stacking up lately caused by killer vitamins. I checked in the U.S. National Poison Data System for their most recent body count of vitamin deaths, but not a single death was caused by a dietary supplement in 2009. Any deaths in 2008? Nope. How about 2007? None. Year after year vitamins seem to harm no one and yet continue to provide remarkable benefits, a situation the drug companies apparently find intolerable.

Just to make certain I did not miss anything, I kept digging. I finally found this (partial) list of deadly killers from the 2003 poison report, and I am not making this up: There were 656 deaths caused by analgesics (painkillers), a total of three deaths were caused by dishwashing detergent, and there was an account of two poor souls who tragically met their end with exposure to some combination of perfume/cologne/aftershave. Talk about a killer fragrance.

Further down the list I found it, the smoking gun, the absolute proof that vitamins are deadly: The average number of deaths each year caused by vitamins over the last few decades is a bit less than one person per year. I wondered, did these people choke on the pills? Did they overdose? There was no further information. Nevertheless, I had to face the awful truth: For every two people that die from using aftershave, one dies from taking vitamins. Now what was I to do? One minute I thought my vitamins were my friends, the next minute it turns out they might be plotting to kill me.

The clear and present danger posed by vitamins must surely account for the NIH panel's recent, urgent pleas to give the Food and Drug Administration (FDA) greater authority and more money to regulate vitamins. It is worth noting that FDA commissioners have testified in Congress that they already have the power to regulate dietary supplements but lack sufficient funds to do so. Not that they don't already have massive gobs of money, but the FDA apparently has other priorities. Not many people realize how expensive it is to fast-track untested and dangerous new drugs and get them to market so the drug ads can begin.

Obviously, we should grant the FDA all the money they need to clamp down on the vitamin menace, but perhaps we shouldn't stop there. We should consider asking the FDA to begin regulating ice cream, double cheeseburgers and deep-fried cookies as soon as possible. Those nutrients are clearly extremely dangerous in the wrong hands.

And hot dogs, of course, are the most dangerous "virtually unregulated" nutrient on the market because of parents who do not have the sense to cut the wieners into little bite-sized pieces before giving them to their children, leaving the kids to choke to death.

I am still puzzled, though, why the panel did not invite some of their colleagues from down the hall at the NIH to their conference, such as Mark Levine, M.D. His groundbreaking research showing increased survival and safety for cancer patients given high-dose intravenous vitamin C, even for advanced late-stage cancer, is so impressive that he has called for a "re-evaluation of vitamin C as a cancer therapy."

Another large NIH study looked at women and heart disease. Cardiovascular deaths dropped 24 percent for women in the study who were taking vitamin E. Incredibly, those who were 65 and older, the very women statistically at a greater risk of heart attacks, saw death rates drop an amazing 49 percent, cutting the risk almost in half.

Can you imagine the media orgy we would see if a drug could perform like that? It would be hailed as a miracle cure, the cost per pill would shoot up to 300 bucks instead of 22 cents, and drug company stocks would soar through the roof.

Luckily for us, vitamins are not patentable, although you can rest assured that Big Pharma scientists are working overtime to tweak vitamin molecules slightly so that they can be patented by Big Pharma lawyers. Watch what happens then; natural vitamins will be illegal and only doctors will prescribe patented vitamin analogs—or, to put it another way, when vitamins are outlawed, only outlaws will have vitamins.

In the meantime, we are cautioned not to exceed the official recommended daily amounts. These official levels are widely recognized to be so absurdly low that ingesting only a fraction less results in the onset of symptoms of degenerative vitamin deficiency diseases.

To be certain, there are three things with which we should concern ourselves when it comes to vitamins, the three factors of quality. Potency: Does the vitamin contain the dosage the packaging says it does? Purity: Is there other junk in there such as fillers and binding agents that may be allergenic? Bioavailability: How well is the body able to disassemble and absorb the vitamins in a particular brand of supplements?

The periodic vitamin attacks from government agencies and others are unwarranted. The safety record of vitamins is unsurpassed. The NIH panel chose to ignore the preponderance of evidence that dietary supplementation is one of the single most important long-term health strategies we have. Beyond that, an avalanche of evidence suggests that therapeutic doses of specific nutrients hold tremendous promise for rescuing millions of people from ill health and chronic disease.

This last point underscores the true danger of taking vitamins: Pharmaceutical companies stand to lose profits from the sale of drugs that are prescribed to treat the symptoms of nutritional deficiency diseases.

As Otto Von Bismark once observed, "Never believe anything in politics until it has been officially denied." Now that the NIH has officially denied that vitamins are beneficial and safe, I know for certain it is time to go back to the kitchen and take my vitamins.

Magnesium Magnificence

Health is the state about which medicine has nothing to say.

W.H. Auden

Everybody gets a headache occasionally, but for chronic migraine sufferers, the headaches can occur frequently and can be totally disabling. Drugs for migraines simply do not work very well, leaving people with chronic migraines ready to try just about anything. Including injections of botulism.

Now blessed by the Food and Drug Administration (FDA) as a treatment for migraines, botulinum toxin is approved for doctors to administer to migraine sufferers who have 15 or more days of headaches per month. The multiple injections are given in the neck muscles and must be repeated each 12 weeks.

Not everyone believes the shots of toxin are a good idea, however, including the American Academy of Neurology (AAN), which in 2008 released guidelines for the clinical use of botulinum toxin preparations. The authors concluded that despite the popularity of using the toxin for headache treatment, it is ineffective for migraine headaches and unlikely to help tension headaches either.

"Based on currently available data, botulinum toxin injections should not be offered to patients with episodic migraine and chronic tension-type headaches," according to AAN pain guidelines author Markus Naumann, M.D., "It is no better than placebo injections for these types of headache."

On the packaging for botulinum toxin is a black-box warning, which is the most serious warning ever required by the FDA short of recalling the drug. This particular black box is a wee bit alarming because it says the toxin can spread from the injection site and cause swallowing and breathing difficulties that may kill you. Other side effects? The most commonly cited reactions are neck pain and—you guessed it—headache.

Chronic headache sufferers may be surprised to learn that there is help available that requires neither a prescription nor a skull-and-cross-bones warning for those who wish to use it: magnesium. Supplementation with this element can minimize or eliminate headaches for many people, and the only side effect is loose stools or diarrhea—but only if too much is taken at once. Not only that, magnesium can significantly reduce pain from fibromyalgia, bring down blood pressure levels, reduce multiple sclerosis relapses, reduce anxiety and depression, relax and repair heart muscle, lower the risk of cognitive decline, prevent leg cramping at night, and promote tooth and bone health—all at the same time.

If magnesium were a drug, it would be one of the most widely prescribed and profitable drugs of all time. Luckily for us it is not patentable, so it is not classified as a drug. It is completely nontoxic, widely available, and inexpensive.

You probably have not heard much about the many miraculous benefits of magnesium, but this is largely due to the apparent unwritten rule among the pharmaceutical companies and government regulatory agencies: If something cannot be patented, there can be no massive profits, and without profits there is no reason to study a substance, much less let the public know about it. And in those cases where a completely natural and vital nutrient works exceptionally well and could actually compete with the sales of pharmaceuticals, stories seem to circulate periodically in the media that the nutrient is useless and ingesting it may be dangerous.

Magnesium is the miracle mineral that does so much and costs so little. The U.S. Department of Agriculture (USDA) reports on its Web site that the majority of adults in the U.S. are deficient in magnesium. Given that USDA scientists' calculations are made using official required daily allowance figures—which are considered ridiculously low by nutrition-conscious clinicians—the actual problem is likely far more widespread than the estimates from the USDA.

"Even a mild deficiency of magnesium can cause increased sensitivity to noise, nervousness, irritability, mental depression, confusion, twitching, trembling, apprehension, and insomnia," writes Mark Sircus, Ac., O.M.D., in his book, *Magnesium—The Ultimate Heart Medicine*. Is it any wonder that ADHD symptoms have been described as virtually identical to the symptoms of chronic magnesium deficiency? The symptoms of movement disorders such as Parkinson's disease are also linked to magnesium deficiency, because magnesium is vital to the production of dopamine.

Foods that provide magnesium include leafy green vegetables, avocados, nuts such as almonds, cashews, pecans and walnuts, whole grains, legumes, figs, and dates. Unfortunately, unless the foods are grown organically, they will contain little magnesium. Standard industrial farming techniques use the standard NPK fertilizers, composed primarily of nitrogen, phosphorous, and potassium. The plant may look healthy enough, but it lacks the vital array of nutrients and micronutrients needed in food for people to maintain good health. Organically grown produce, on the other hand, is grown in topsoil constantly replenished with compost that supplies nutrients such as magnesium.

"However, if you are suffering from the following symptoms you may need supplemental magnesium: muscle twitches, tics, or spasms; 'Charlie horse' (the muscle spasm that occurs when you stretch your legs); insomnia or restless sleep; stress; back pain; headaches, cluster headaches, migraines; stiff and aching muscles; bones and joints that need continued chiropractic treatment; weakness; hypoglycemia; diabetes; nervousness; hyperactivity; high blood pressure; osteoporosis; PMS; constipation; angina; kidney stones; aging; depression; heart attack; irregular heartbeat; attention deficit disorder; aggressive behavior; chronic fatigue syndrome; stroke; anxiety; confusion, muscle weakness; hiccups; seizures; high-strung; exhaustion from exercise," writes Carolyn Dean, M.D., N.D., in her book, *The Miracle of Magnesium*.

Imagine the tall stack of drug prescriptions needed to treat all of the preceding symptoms, not to mention the cost. Then there is the long list of adverse effects possibly caused by each drug, some requiring additional drugs to mitigate the adverse symptoms they cause.

Obviously, many of the health disorders listed above have confounding factors beyond magnesium deficiency. Every individual is unique, has a unique health history, and has a genetic heritage that may predispose him or her to certain health problems. But considering that magnesium is vital for the proper functioning of each and every cell, as well as being a requirement for the correct metabolic function of more than 350 enzymes in the body, evaluating magnesium levels should be the first order of business in a health assessment. In other words, it makes sense to rule out magnesium deficiency before diagnosing any one of a long list of health disorders whose symptoms overlap with magnesium deficiency.

And it is all too easy to become magnesium deficient. Mental stress, menstruation, a diet high in processed foods, high salt intake—as well as alcohol, caffeine, tobacco, and many prescription drugs—all cause the loss of magnesium through the urine.

The official required daily allowance of magnesium gives only the absolute minimum level needed to avoid deficiency symptoms, currently set at 300 milligrams per day for women and 400 milligrams per day for men. Magnesium citrate and magnesium malate are formulations of the mineral considered by many to be the best tolerated and most bioavailable. Since the body easily eliminates excess magnesium, it is safe to start supplementing with the required daily allowance and increase the dosage each day to "oral tolerance," or a dosage level that causes the bowels to be a bit loose.

However, for many people who are severely depleted of magnesium, the oral tolerance dosage is insufficient to build up magnesium to healthy levels. Luckily, magnesium is easily absorbed transdermally, or through the skin.

"There are many advantages to transdermal magnesium therapy, since the gastrointestinal tract is avoided altogether and there is no laxative effect. Next to intravenous magnesium administration, transdermal therapy provides a greater amount of magnesium to be absorbed than even the best tolerated oral supplements, and can restore intracellular concentrations in a matter of weeks rather than the months required for oral supplementation," according to the Weston A. Price Foundation on its Web site.

Many people use Epsom salts without realizing they are soaking in magnesium sulfate or engaging in transdermal therapy. Magnesium sulfate can help a variety of problems, but there is another formulation that is more effective and longer lasting because it is readily absorbed deeply into the cells: magnesium chloride. Magnesium chloride is available as powdery flakes ready for adding to bathwater and also in a liquid form called magnesium oil, which can be spread directly on the skin or poured into the bath. This is not really an oil at all, but a supersaturated concentration of magnesium chloride derived from seawater that feels slippery like oil. Magnesium supplements and Epsom salts are widely available at drugstores and health food stores, but magnesium chloride flakes and magnesium oil are not, so they must be ordered online through sources on the Internet.

Achieving sufficient intracellular magnesium in the body may seem a bit troublesome and transdermal magnesium therapy, unorthodox, but doing so has the potential to radically improve one's health today as well as prevent a surprisingly wide array of health challenges in future years.

The War Against Vitamin D

A vitamin is a substance that makes you ill if you don't eat it.

Albert Szent-Györgyi

The most recent battle in the ongoing war against vitamins involves vitamin D, and major casualties have once again been sustained on the battlefield of American public health. The newest weapon of mass health destruction unleashed by the drug companies and their government regulatory buddies is a new set of guidelines for vitamin D dosage and safe upper limits.

Safe upper limits, are you kidding me? First, let us set the record straight on the safety of vitamins. "Over half of the U.S. population takes daily nutritional supplements. Even if each of those people took only one single tablet daily, that makes 155,000,000 doses per day, for a total of nearly 57 billion doses annually. Since many persons take more than just one vitamin or mineral tablet, actual consumption is considerably higher, and the safety of nutritional supplements is all the more remarkable," reported the Orthomolecular Medicine news service. "If nutritional supplements are allegedly so 'dangerous,' as the FDA and news media so often claim, then where are the bodies?"

To get an idea of the threat posed to Big Pharma by vitamin D, consider this summary of vitamin D attributes posted on the Web site of the Vitamin D Council, written by health consumer advocate Bill Sardi: "There is not a chronic disease—ranging from heart disease to cancer, from the flu to tuberculosis, from diabetes to schizophrenia, from rickets in infants to osteoporosis among older women—that is not exaggerated by shortages of vitamin D. Vitamin D deficiency is a universal factor in all disease states, even for populations living in sunny areas where natural vitamin D production is expected to be high."

For years clinicians have been pushing for higher vitamin D intake recommendations because of the avalanche of research published in the past ten years linking vitamin D deficiency to a startling array of health disorders. An adequate intake of vitamin D3 activates the immune system and helps restore the body's ability to heal.

Clearly, the authority to write vitamin guidelines with the potential to positively transform the health of millions of people presents a tremendous opportunity. So who is given this power in our country? It is the Institutes of Medicine (IOM), through its Food and Nutrition Board. The IOM is one of those quasi-governmental bodies with enormous political and economic power over our daily lives that is run by political appointees from the medical industry.

On the IOM's Web site we read, "The Institutes of Medicine is an independent, nonprofit organization that works outside of government to provide unbiased and authoritative advice to decision makers and the public." The Web site also states, "The Institutes of Medicine serves as adviser to the nation to improve health."

For those familiar with the IOM's role in vitamin recommendations, a more accurate description might read more like this: The Institutes of Medicine works to improve the health of Big Pharma companies by ensuring the profitability of drug sales for a wide range of health disorders resulting from poor nutrition and vitamin deficiencies.

Glenville Jones, Ph.D., is one of the "unbiased" appointees to the fourteen-member "expert" vitamin D panel. Jones also happens to be an advisor to a drug company developing a "vitamin D analog." (A vitamin analog is a vitamin molecule tweaked in the laboratory just enough to make it patentable.) The company is testing its vitamin D wannabe on patients with chronic kidney disorder; not surprisingly, it helps people get well.

Jones is quoted as saying most people "probably don't have vitamin D deficiency." This suggests one of two things, either Dr. Jones has not read a single thing about vitamin D in the past ten years, or else he knows all about it and wants to keep the importance of vitamin D a secret.

Most vitamin D experts express a point of view that is pretty much the opposite of Jones' opinion. Michael F. Holick, M.D., Ph.D., from the Boston University School of Medicine said, "We estimate that vitamin D deficiency is the most common medical condition in the world."

"Because vitamin D is so cheap and so clearly reduces all-cause mortality, I can say this with great certainty: Vitamin D represents the single most cost-effective medical intervention in the United States," said Greg Plotnikoff, M.D., Medical Director at Abbott Northwestern Hospital in Minneapolis.

"I would recommend that every patient, every person in America get their vitamin D checked, because so many people are low and the ramifications of having low vitamin D are so severe," said Richard Honaker, M.D., family practice physician.

The Food and Nutrition Board did increase the required daily allowance marginally. The new recommendation is that 600 IU (International Units) per day is plenty; however, anything over 4,000 IU is unsafe. Meanwhile, experts at the Vitamin D Council and Harvard Medical School recommend in the range of 1,000 to 5,000 IU every day for optimum health. It is also reported that up to 10,000 IU can safely be taken without a doctor's supervision.

The news media, for some reason, treated the miniscule change in the vitamin guidelines as a vitamin D health scare. A headline in *The Wall Street Journal* asked, "Can Too Much Vitamin D Be Hazardous to Your Health?" And CBS warned, "Vitamin D Report Shocker: High Doses Unnecessary, Risky."

As the war on vitamins continues, you may notice a consistent strategy emerging. Stories crop up in the media claiming that vitamins are worthless but, on the other hand, are terribly dangerous. Pressure is exerted at the highest levels to maintain official daily vitamin doses at absurdly low levels, effectively preventing many people from experiencing the health benefits of vitamin supplementation. Finally, patented vitamin analogs are made available as prescription drugs at outrageously high prices. And since these "new drugs" closely mimic the real vitamin molecule, people experience great benefits, making profits soar.

Fortify yourself against Big Pharma's war on vitamins by finding a good source of natural vitamins. You will also need sources of information about vitamins that are not generated by Big Pharma and its war propaganda machine—which seems to have infiltrated more than a few government agencies.

Weighing in on Obesity and Inflammation

Imprisoned in every fat man, a thin one is wildly signaling to be let out.
Cyril Connolly

Until recently I was fairly neutral about the whole extra weight/overweight trend in our country. As a chiropractor, when I look at a heavy person I see mechanical stress in the joints and the spine caused by the extra weight and the resulting risk to the knees, ankles, hips and vertebrae of wearing out prematurely and developing arthritis.

Beyond those considerations, though, I was never overly concerned with people's extra weight—that is, until I learned that people who are chronically overweight suffer chronic inflammation in the body, which is definitely not good news. We'll have some good news in a minute, but first a few fast facts on fat.

The buildup of adipose tissue, or fat, in the body is, without exception, accompanied by a low-level inflammatory response of the immune system that just won't quit—as long as the fat stores remain. Inflammation is the same underlying condition present in numerous chronic diseases, including type II diabetes, Alzheimer's disease, and heart disease. Scientists have observed that inflammatory immune cells migrate to fat tissue in overweight persons, even in the absence of physical injury.

"Findings in adult humans and in animals suggest that the inflammatory status associated with the increase of fat mass may be involved in the pathogenetic pathways of obesity complications," according to the January 2006 issue of the journal *Pediatrics*. Translated, this means that having excessive stores of fat in the body triggers the expression of genes that create inflammation. Why? Scientists do not know why inflammation is triggered, but we do know quite a bit about inflammation.

Inflammation is a normal, potentially life-saving response by the immune system. For example, an inflammatory response is a necessary step in recovering from physical bodily injury. Special immune cells in the body are activated, whose job is to produce swelling (this helps "wall off" the affected area by closing vessel drainage), turn up the heat (which makes it more difficult for any microbes to infect the host), and carry out major house cleaning and repair (with special cells that take apart and recycle human cellular tissue).

Although normal healing for just about every type of physical injury or immune challenge requires some level of an acute inflammatory reaction and process, chronic inflammation, the kind found in excess fat tissue, is the same kind of inflammation observed in chronic illness.

For a long time scientists have argued back and forth with the classic chicken-and-egg debate when it comes to the link between being overweight and its association with a growing list of health disorders. Which came first, the asthma or the obesity? Does cancer result from obesity, or are obese people just genetically predisposed to cancer? We simply do not know for sure, but understanding that inflammation shows up where extra fat is stored may emerge as an important key to our understanding. To the extent that chronic inflammation can be reduced or prevented altogether, chronic health disorders associated with inflammation may also be reduced or prevented.

The number of obese adults and children has risen nearly 50 percent in only 20 years. Nearly a third of adults and fully one-fourth of children are now clinically obese, defined as a body mass index of 30 or greater.

"Overweight and obesity are both labels for ranges of weight that are greater than what is generally considered healthy for a given height," according to the Centers for Disease Control's Web site.

The list of serious health problems associated with being overweight and obese is significant and daunting. As we've already seen, heart disease is on the list, including heart attack, congestive heart failure, sudden cardiac death, angina or chest pain, high blood pressure, and high blood triglycerides, according to the Surgeon General.

Other problems include type II diabetes, asthma, stroke, gallstones, liver disease, arthritis, gout, infertility in men, and irregular menstruation in women. Cancer is also associated with obesity. For women it is cancer of the uterus, gallbladder, cervix, ovaries, breasts, and colon. For men the higher risk is for colorectal and prostate cancer.

For children who grow up obese, certain effects may be permanent, such as smaller lung size due to the mechanical stress and space limitations of added mass within the chest cavity during the growth years.

"We know that obesity in children has a carry-over effect to adulthood," says Ramin Alemzadeh, M.D., Professor of Pediatrics at the Medical College of Wisconsin. "But diabetes is not the only issue related to childhood obesity. Obese children may have greater difficulty with high blood pressure, high cholesterol levels, orthopedic problems, sleeping habits, as well as self-esteem and peer relationships," he said.

Doing its part to trim the growing American waistline, the federal government has gotten involved, especially targeting obesity in children. School administrations, already stretched to the limit meeting other requirements, must now provide wellness programs. In some school districts this has created the irony of wellness lifestyle lectures being delivered by teachers whose physical appearance suggests that living a healthy lifestyle is very unfamiliar territory.

To be sure, there are many factors that may lead to obesity in children, not the least of which is obesity in parents. Whether this is a genetic predisposition or the result of a lifestyle learned from parents is another question that has yet to be answered.

Other potential causes of obesity are environmental. By environmental we mean everything that makes its way into the body, including the food we eat, the air we breathe, and the water we drink. It also includes the difference between healthy habits and self-destructive habits, such as exercising versus exercise avoidance, and positive versus negative thinking. To this list we must add hormone dysregulation caused by exposure to chemical hormone disrupters, such as pesticides, plastics, detergents, and heavy metals, to name a few.

Not surprisingly, the discovery that inflammation accompanies obesity has some members of the medical community reflexively reaching for their prescription pads to prescribe anti-inflammatory medications, with the aim of blocking the inflammatory processes triggered by being overweight. Unfortunately, this strategy carries with it numerous unintended and undesirable side effects, because anti-inflammatory drugs are known to suppress multiple beneficial cellular functions throughout the body and greatly increase the risk of cardiovascular disorders.

"Investigators saw an increase in myocardial infarctions, stroke, and cardiovascular death in patients taking all of these NSAIDs [nonsteroidal anti-inflammatory drugs]," reported the online *Medscape Today* in January 2011.

Various surgical methods for achieving weight loss, such as gastric bypass, have become quite common and can be effective, although their effectiveness is primarily due to the necessity of drastically changing one's eating habits following the surgery.

Unfortunately, surgical solutions for gaining control of weight also carry the risk of serious side effects. These include surgical complications, excessive bleeding, leaks in the gastrointestinal system, infections, bowel obstruction, hernias, gallstones, ulcers, vomiting, stomach perforation, weight regain, deep vein thrombosis, blood clots in the lungs, and malnutrition, according to the Mayo Clinic on its Web site.

The good news is that millions of people have accomplished natural, permanent weight loss without resorting to drugs or surgery. The methods range widely, none of them are easy, and all require a serious commitment to make lifestyle changes. Heavily advertised special diets, diet medications, and liquid nutrition programs are doomed to fail for the majority of people who try them. Ask someone you know who has successfully changed their life through significant weight loss and you'll likely hear about radical transformations in their relationship to food, upgrading the quality of the food they eat, and getting disciplined about regular exercise.

Self-health strategies are the safest and most effective means to shed extra pounds, thereby reducing systemic inflammation as well as the risk of serious health problems now and in the future. In the words of philosopher Robert Ingersoll, "In nature there are neither rewards nor punishments—there are only consequences."

Taking Life One Day at a Time

The man who has lived the longest is not he who has spent the greatest number of years, but he who has had the greatest sensibility of life.

Jean-Jacques Rousseau

"Congratulations Mrs. Jones, your 87-year-old husband has a new heart, one new lung and a couple of new kidneys. The procedure was difficult but 100 percent successful. We did a great job."

"But my husband died on the operating room table!"

"Oh yes, that was a pity. We are very sorry, but as you can see from this hospital bill, we did absolutely everything we could think of. Speaking of the bill, the total amount you owe us is $178,542. Will that be cash, check, or credit card?"

Here in America we have a solid tradition of treating old age as a disease and viewing death as the ultimate enemy. We can, we must, we shall fight death! To the, um, death! Even if it kills us! And it does. How amazing is it that roughly 80 percent of the money spent on all the medical care in a person's life occurs in the last few weeks of life?

"The four stages of life are infancy, childhood, adolescence and obsolescence," said Art Linkletter. He was joking of course, but it does seem that people who believe old age means you become sick and disabled will likely end up that way. If good health and long life are our goals, we would be wise to study people who live long, healthy lives.

At times, the world is enriched with an individual who lives a long, healthy life and becomes a legend in his own time. I was nine when just such a man moved in next door, my grandfather Bert.

He was born in 1881 in Pennsylvania. Bert climbed the ladder of success one rung at a time, starting at a young age and rising over the years from office boy all the way to vice president of a farm implement company in St. Paul, Minnesota. When the Great Depression hit, though, his company was wiped off the map, and so was his career. Undaunted, the resilient optimist that he was, Bert declared, "We might starve, but we won't freeze!" as he and my grandmother Isabel moved their four children west with them to California.

Grandpa was a jokester and folk philosopher. He joked and laughed right up to the last day of his 99 years, just months shy of 100. "It's a terrible thing getting old," he used to say, "but it beats the alternative!" That was the closest thing to a complaint Bert ever uttered about growing old. He was a living example of how you needn't become aged just because you are getting older. When people would ask how he was doing, he would sometimes answer, "I've still got all my marbles, but I think they're rattling around a bit in there!"

Of course, Bert's excellent health during his long life did not necessarily stem from ten decades of a strict health-food diet. When I was ten he explained to me about balanced meals, "Hold the hot dog in one hand and the glass of root beer in the other." Significantly though, he would often describe the foods he ate in great quantities in all his early years: farm-fresh food. In those days, there was no fuss over whether food was grown organically. Locally grown, farm-fresh vegetables, dairy, and meats when Bert was a boy were all free of antibiotics, hormones, pesticides and herbicides, and other chemicals that are increasingly linked to chronic health disorders today.

Bert was able to get up and get around doing the things he enjoyed up to the very end of his days, especially tending his roses. He moved around more easily than many people twenty and even thirty years his junior and never seemed preoccupied with old age. He advised us all to "stay on the sunny side of life," and "take life one day at a time."

He loved to walk, and he did so nearly every day. A very long dirt road used to connect our old ranch property to the main road—that is, until the housing development bulldozed its way into our valley. Bert would walk down that long dirt drive in the morning to pick up the newspaper and bring it home and then later walk back down and carry the day's bundle of mail back up the hill.

Bert was full of practical advice. "Sleep when you're tired, and get up when you're hungry," he would say, and, "Stay away from medical doctors!" He followed his own advice and could count on one hand the number of times he was prescribed drugs in all his years. I am told that the average senior citizen today swallows a handful of drugs every single day.

Somehow a belief has crept into our culture that growing old means growing feeble and ill and that drugs and surgery will likely be needed just to stay alive. When survival is granted supreme importance, quality of life goes out the window. Now I'm not suggesting that allopathic medical doctors created this situation, but doctors do seem to expect aging patients to become miserably dysfunctional as a natural course of events. Perhaps this is because the healthy seniors are staying away from medical offices in droves, so doctors never have a chance to meet them and be exposed to healthy people with 8 or 9 decades under their belts still living drug free.

Setting aside the question of whether or not seniors benefit from taking a dozen pills a day, it is an enormous burden to pay for all this medical stuff, Medicare or no. The ever-shifting rules of engagement with Medicare make me think we should change the name to "Medi-*don't-care*."

Seriously though, if you are interested in staying young and healthy while growing old, you should make a point to talk to some of the healthy senior citizens walking around your town. Find out what their secret is to a long and happy life. Chances are they are aware of Mark Twain's secret just as Grandpa Bert was, "Let us endeavor so to live that when we come to die even the undertaker will be sorry."

Healthy Teeth, Healthy Spine,
Healthy Heart

He's the best physician that knows the worthlessness of the most medicines.
Benjamin Franklin

Did you know that one of the best ways to keep your heart healthy is to keep your teeth healthy? It appears that your dentist's advice about daily tooth brushing and flossing may be more universally effective than taking the pills your cardiologist prescribes, according to a study published in the May 2010 *British Medical Journal* (BMJ).

The same BMJ issue featured a report that statins, a class of drugs used to lower cholesterol, one of the largest-selling prescription medications in history, could be harming more people than it helps. The study found that statistically, for every person whose heart disease is eased by a statin drug, at least two people suffered substantial harm to their health. These newly created problems include kidney failure, serious muscle pain and damage, cataracts, and liver damage.

According to the study, for every 10,000 women taking statins, there were 3 percent fewer cases of heart disease. Of course, the category "heart disease" includes a broad range of problems, from mild arrhythmia to actual heart attack, so a 3 percent reduction in the incidence of heart disease does not mean 3 percent fewer heart attacks.

And now consider the collateral damage observed in the study: 23 cases of acute kidney failure, 74 cases of liver damage, 39 cases of serious muscle dysfunction, and 307 cases of cataracts. The final score in the study was 271 people helped, 443 harmed. The odds of gaining a benefit from taking statin drugs appears to be below 3 chances in 100, whereas the chance for harm is better than 4 in 100.

"Cholesterol is not the major culprit in heart disease or any disease," according to heart specialist Don Rosedale, M.D. "Using the same conventional medical thinking that is being used for cholesterol would lead one to believe that doctors should reduce the risk of Alzheimer's disease by taking out everybody's brain," said Rosedale in a report published on Mercola.com.

"Statins lower cholesterol by suppressing the activity of an enzyme in the liver involved in the production of cholesterol," according to Julian Whitaker, M.D., of the renowned Whitaker Wellness Center. "But this enzyme has multiple functions, including the synthesis of coenzyme Q10. CoQ10 is a key player in the metabolic processes that energize our cells. No wonder statin users suffer from fatigue, muscle pain and weakness, and even heart failure—the cells are simply running out of juice.

"The second most frequent adverse effects of statins are problems with memory, mood, suicidal behavior, and neurological issues. Other common complaints include sexual dysfunction and liver and digestive problems. Symptoms range from minor (achiness, forgetfulness) to serious (complete but temporary amnesia, permanent memory loss) to lethal (congestive heart failure, rhabdomyolysis or complete muscle breakdown). One statin drug, Baycol, was taken off the market a few years ago after it caused dozens of deaths from rhabdomyolysis. Several studies have also linked statin drugs with an increased risk of cancer," said Whitaker.

Are you taking a statin drug? If so, did your doctor mention to you the serious health risks involved? After nearly two decades of accumulated scientific evidence showing little benefit and much evidence of significant harm, a fair question to ask is why do so many doctors still prescribe so many statin drugs?

"A mistake that is rarely made in the hard-core sciences such as physics seems to be frequently made in medicine," Dr. Rosedale explained. "This is confusing correlation with cause. There may be a weak correlation of elevated cholesterol with heart attacks; however this does not mean it is the cholesterol that caused the heart attack. Certainly gray hair is correlated with getting older; however one could hardly say that the gray hair caused one to get old."

According to Dr. Whitaker, "No matter what you've been led to believe, a high cholesterol level is not a reliable sign of an impending heart attack. In fact, growing numbers of experts question whether cholesterol matters at all. As for statin drugs, for most of the 40-plus million Americans recommended to take them for the rest of their lives, they're an ineffective, expensive, side effect–riddled fraud."

What about low-dose aspirin for prevention of cardiovascular disease? Interestingly, there is a big difference of opinion between British and U.S. cardiologists. In both countries, aspirin is recognized to help prevent a second heart attack, but not for preventing the first one.

A study in the April 2010 *British Medical Journal* on low-dose aspirin concluded, "In primary prevention, however, use of low dose aspirin is unlicensed in the United Kingdom, and published evidence does not support the assumption that the benefits clearly outweigh the harms. So the routine practice of starting patients on such treatment for primary prevention of cardiovascular disease should be abandoned."

Okay, so maybe aspirin doesn't really do much good, but it is harmless, right? Maybe not. A study in the *Journal of the American Medical Association* March 2010 cautioned, "Any effect of aspirin on cardiovascular events needs to be balanced against the potential for harm. Although the numbers were small, the trial results suggested an increased incidence of major hemorrhage and gastrointestinal ulcer, although not severe anemia, in the aspirin group, and more participants in the aspirin group than in the placebo group had fatal intracranial adverse events."

In addition to statin drugs and aspirin, several types of pharmaceuticals are prescribed to lower blood pressure. Each type of drug alters the body's biochemical pathways, and each drug comes with its own impressive list of potential adverse effects.

One class of drugs used to reduce blood pressure, beta-blockers, was withdrawn from use in the United Kingdom in 2006 following a review of safety studies that showed an actual increase in the risk of heart attack and stroke compared to other drugs, as well as an increased risk of up to 50 percent for developing type 2 diabetes. Side effects of beta-blockers include cold hands and feet, weakness, dizziness, dry mouth and skin, shortness of breath, memory loss, confusion, depression, and impotence. Despite of all the problems associated with this class of drugs, beta-blockers are still widely prescribed in the United States.

How about calcium channel blockers, another popular antihypertensive? As long ago as 1966 the National Institutes of Health warned, "Postmenopausal women who take calcium channel blockers have twice the risk of developing breast cancer than other women." Calcium channel blockers may also cause heart palpitations, swollen ankles, constipation, dizziness, and headache.

Another antihypertensive class of drugs is ACE inhibitors. Women who are pregnant reportedly should avoid this drug altogether because of the great risk of birth defects. Additionally, ACE inhibitors are associated with kidney failure (particularly for diabetics), allergic reactions, skin rash, loss of taste, and potassium imbalance.

Yet another class of antihypertensives is diuretic drugs, which are often prescribed in combination with other antihypertensives. Side effects include dizziness, nausea, digestive difficulties, muscle pain, skin rash, impotence, and for long-term users, gout.

For people who have naturally low or normal blood pressure, there is a clear positive association with greater cardiovascular health. But how about the people whose blood pressure is lowered with a drug or combination of drugs? Do they experience better heart health? We simply do not know. The assumption is that it does improve cardiovascular health, but no scientific study has ever taken up that question. The bottom line is that drugs for lowering blood pressure are among the most widely prescribed drugs in the modern world, yet there is no clinical evidence that these drugs are doing anybody any good.

Is your doctor up to speed on the down side of blood-pressure-lowering drugs? In an article entitled "What Your Doctor May Not Tell You About Blood Pressure" from the *Virginia Hopkins Health Watch* newsletter, John Lee, M.D., wrote, "I believe—and there is plenty of research to support me—that these drugs have just as good a chance of killing you as the high blood pressure does, especially if you don't really need them."

Dr. Whitaker's advice: "As you can see, we need to shift away from this myopic focus on statin drugs and lowering cholesterol, and take a more holistic view. Folks, you don't need statins—you need a program that addresses all the known risk factors for heart attack, stroke, and other cardiovascular disorders."

Cardiovascular disease is now widely recognized as a lifestyle disease, meaning that many heart health–building steps are available without prescription. These include daily physical, mental, and spiritual exercise, organic nutrition, vitamin/mineral supplementation, plenty of rest, and pure drinking water.

What else can you do? See your chiropractor. The *Journal of Human Hypertension* in March 2007 highlighted research using an upper cervical chiropractic adjustment that can lower blood pressure and keep it low in patients with cervical spine misalignment. "This procedure has the effect of not one, but two blood-pressure medications given in combination. And it seems to be adverse-event free. We saw no side effects and no problems," according to George Bakris, M.D., study leader and director of the University of Chicago hypertension center.

Healthy teeth, healthy spine, healthy heart? For those wanting to improve their heart health without the multiple risks and unknown benefits of medication, it could be that chiropractors and dentists have compelling advice: Get your spine checked and adjusted periodically, and brush and floss your teeth daily.

Bibliography

I have purposely used limited references within the text instead of footnotes so that the reader may concentrate on the nonmainstream information and ideas presented in the book with less distraction. The predominant ideas in the field of natural healing are based on timeless healing traditions, common sense, and biological principles that are independent of reference sources. Documentation of the extraordinary and abysmal failure of modern allopathic medicine is, in 2012, widely published and well known outside the mainstream allopathic medical community.

For those who are interested in further research into the major ideas expressed in this book, I recommend several informative books.

Stephanie Cave, M.D. and Deborah Mitchell, *What your Doctor May Not Tell You about Children's Vaccinations*. New York: Hachette Book Group, 2001.

Paul Connett, Ph.D., et al, *The Case Against Fluoride: How Hazardous Waste Ended Up in Our Drinking Water, and the Bad Science and Powerful Politics That Keeps It There*. White River Jct., VT: Chelsea Green Publishing Company, 2010.

Harris L. Coulter and Barbara Loe Fisher, *A Shot in the Dark*. New York: Harcourt, Brace, Jovanovich, 1985.

Cynthia Cournoyer, *What About Immunizations? Exposing the Vaccine Philosophy*. Grants Pass, OR: Better Books Publishing, 2010.

Carolyn Dean, M.D., N.D., *Death by Modern Medicine*. Belleville, Ontario: Matrix Verite Media, 2005.

Carolyn Dean, M.D., N.D., *The Magnesium Miracle*. New York: Random House, 2003.

Catherine J.M. Diodati, M.A., *Immunization History, Ethics, Law and Health*. Windsor, Ontario: Integral Aspects, Inc., 1999.

Mayer Eisenstein, M.D., J.D., M.P.H., *Don't Vaccinate! Before You Educate*. Chicago: CMI Press, 2002.

Joel Fuhrman, M.D., *Fasting and Eating for Health—A Medical Doctor's Program for Conquering Disease*. New York: St. Martin's Press, 1995.

Charlotte Gerson and Morton Walker, D.P.M., *The Gerson Therapy*. New York: Kensington Publishing Corporation, 2001.

Louise Kuo Habakus, M.A. and Mary Holland, J.D., *Vaccine Epidemic*. New York: Skyhorse Publishing, 2011.

Mark Hyman, M.D., *The Ultramind Solution*. New York: Simon and Schuster, 2008.

Walene James, *Immunization—The Reality Behind the Myth*. Westport, CT: Greenwood Publishing Group, Inc., 1995.

Joel M. Kaufman, PhD., *Malignant Medical Myths*. West Conshohocken, PA: Infinity Publishing Co., 2006.

David Kirby, *Evidence of Harm—Mercury in Vaccines and the Autism Epidemic: A Medical Controversy*. New York: St. Martin's Press, 2005.

Beth Lambert and Victoria Kobliner, M.S., R.D., *A Compromised Generation—The Epidemic of Chronic Illness in America's Children*. Boulder, CO: Sentient Publications, 2010.

William Joel Meggs, M.D., Ph.D., *The Inflammation Cure*. New York: McGraw-Hill, 2004.

Robert S. Mendelsohn, M.D., *Confessions of a Medical Heretic*. Chicago: Contemporary Books, 1979.

Robert S. Mendelsohn, M.D., *How to Raise a Healthy Child...In Spite of Your Doctor*. New York: Random House, 1984.

Ray Moynihan and Alan Cassels, *Selling Sickness*. New York: Nation Books, 2005.

Dan Olmsted and Mark Blaxill, *The Age of Autism—Mercury, Medicine, and a Man-Made Epidemic.* New York: St. Martin's Press, 2010.

Eric Plasker, D.C., *The 100-Year Lifestyle.* Avon, MA: F&W Publications Company, 2007.

Byron J. Richards, *Fight for Your Health—Exposing the FDA's Betrayal of America.* Tucson, AZ: Truth In Wellness, LLC.

John Robbins, *Reclaiming Our Health.* Tiburon, CA: H.J. Kramer, 1996.

Andrew W. Saul, Ph.D., *Fire Your Doctor! How to Be Independently Healthy.* Laguna Beach, CA: Basic Health Publications, Inc., 2005.

Viera Scheibner, Ph.D., *Vaccination—100 Years of Orthodox Research shows that Vaccines Represent a Medical Assault on the Immune System.* Victoria, Australia: Australia Print Group, 1993.

Sherri Tenpenny, D.O., *Saying No to Vaccines—A Resource Guide for All Ages.* Cleveland, OH: NMA Media Press, 2008.

Andrew Wakefield, *Callous Disregard, Autism and Vaccines, The Truth Behind a Tragedy.* New York: Skyhorse Publishing, 2011

Index

A

ABC News, coverage of vitamins, 185

ACE inhibitors, 208

ADA. *See* American Dental Association.

ADD. *See* attention deficit disorder.

ADHD. *See* attention deficit hyperactivity disorder.

Advertising, drug, 62, 161–4

Advisory Committee on Immunization Practice (ACIP), 30, 32

Agency for Toxic Substances and Disease Registry, 179

Alcabes, Philp, 51

Allopathy, 63, 68, 100, 134, 137, 204

Alzheimer's, and flu shots, 95

AMA. *See* American Medical Association.

American Academy of Neurology (AAN), 189–90

American Academy of Pediatrics (AAP), 128–9, 131

American Cancer Society (ACS), 85, 171, 172, 174

Breast Health Awareness Program, 174

American Dental Association (ADA), 177

American Institute of Ultrasound in Medicine, 116

American Journal of Public Health, 10, 87

American Medical Association (AMA), 21, 33, 88, 99–100, 116

American Psychiatric Association (APA), 124

American Social Health Association, 81

Antibiotics, and asthma, 137

misuse of, 70, 150

Antidepressant drugs, 167

Antipsychotic drugs, 148

Antivirals, 52

Archives of Internal Medicine, 91

Aspirin, 207

Association of American Physicians and Surgeons, 83

Asthma, 133–8, 199

and foods to avoid, 137

environmental causes of, 136-7

AstraZeneca Pharmaceuticals, 172

Attention deficit disorder (ADD),
124–7

Attention deficit hyperactivity
disorder (ADHD), 124–7, 140

Auden, W.H., 189

*Australian and New Zealand Journal of
Public Health*, 181

Avian flu, 152–6

Ayoub, David, M.D., 31

B

Bailar, John, M.D., 171

Bakris, George, M.D., 99

Baughman, Fred, Jr., M.D., 125

Beech, Beverley Lawrence, 117

Berkelhamer, Jay. M.D., 145

Besser, Richard, Dr., 148

Beta-blockers, 207-8

Big Pharma, 7, 25, 28, 37, 43, 46, 64,
121, 131, 148, 149, 162, 166-7,
169, 173, 175, 195, 197

Blood pressure, 98–99, 101, 109,
207–8
and ACE inhibitors, 208
and beta-blockers, 207
and calcium channel blockers, 208
and diuretics, 208

Bohr, Niels, 120

Breast cancer, 170–5
mammograms and, 173–4
risk factors, 173
thermal imaging, 174

Breast Cancer Action, 173

Breast Cancer Fund, 173

Brecht, Bertolt, 115

Breggin, Peter, M.D., 127

British Medical Journal, 71, 100, 130,
164, 205, 207

Buckley, Sarah, M.D., 112

Bureau of Radiological Health, 118

Bush, George W., 119

Business Week, 100

C

Caesar, Julius, 24

Calcium channel blockers, 208

California, fluoridation of water,
177, 179

Canadian Association of Dental
Research, 179

Canadian Medical Association Journal,
12

Cancer, breast, 170–5
chances of, 171
and obesity, 200

Cannell, John Jacob, M.D., 93

Cardiovascular disease, 128-32, 205-
9

Catalano, Robert, 152

CBS News, coverage of Vitamin D,
196
coverage of swine flu, 49–50

Cell function, 58–61
abnormal, 60
normal, 59

Centers for Disease Control (CDC),
9–10, 29–31, 49–55, 73-76, 81,
83-86, 91, 93, 96, 148, 178, 200
Pink Book, 9-10

Cervarix, 84, 87

Cervical cancer, 84–87

Cesarean sections, 30, 109, 112–13

Cheraskin, Emanuel, M.D., 34, 62,
66

Chest Journal, 77

Chicken pox, 15, 17. *See also* vaccination.

Chickens and avian flu, 152–6

Chiropractic, 20–21
and ADHD, 126
and asthma, 136–7
and blood pressure, 99, 101
and earaches, 71
general benefits of, 99-101
and heart health, 209

Cholesterol levels, in children,
128–32

and cholesterol-lowering drugs, 129–32
Chronic disease, 6, 64, 67
    preventing, 68
Chronic inflammation, 198–201
Cicero, 176
CIN, 85
Circumcision, 110–11
CNN Money Web site, 173
Cold medicine, 143–6
Colds, 143–6
Collaborative on Health and the Environment, 135
Committee on Unproven Methods of Cancer Management, 172–3
Connolly, Cyril, 198
Consumer Healthcare Products Association, 143
CoQ10, 131, 206

D
Dean, Carolyn. M.D., N.D., 191
Dean, Trendley, D.D.S., 177
Dental health, 205–9
    and fluoride, 176–83
Department of Agriculture (USDA), 191
Department of Health and Human Services, 69, 179
Desoto, Dr. Joseph, 88
Dickson, Robert, M.D., 183
Direct-to-consumer (DTC) drug advertising, 161-4
Discover Magazine, 85
Disease management, 6–8, 43
Diseases, number of, 58
    successful treatment of, 67
Disraeli, Benjamin, 69
Diuretics, 208
Dogma, 44–46
    of medicine, 46
Donegan, Jayne, M.D., 12
Drug companies, 6, 96, 148-51, 168
Drug Enforcement Agency, 127

Drugs, 59, 123–7,147–151
    advertising, 62, 161–4, 167
    antidepressants, 167
    antipsychotic, 148
    cholesterol, 128–32
    and colds, 143–6
    definition, 26
    fast-track approval, 166
    for insomnia, 165–9
    overdoses, 148
    overprescribed, 124, 126,148
    prescription, 2, 6, 147-51, 161–4
    safety, 47, 126–7, 129–32, 134, 148, 167, 185
    side effects, 127, 167–9, 190, 205–8
DuPont, 174

E
Earaches, 69-72
    and chiropractic, 71
    wait-and-see prescription, 70
Earth Island Journal, 177
Eddy, David, M.D., Ph.D., 100
Edison, Thomas, 102
Emesis, definition, 105
Environmental Protection Agency (EPA), 60, 95
Environmental toxins, 4–5
EPA. *See* Environmental Protection Agency.
Epsom salts, 192
Epstein, Samuel, M.D., 173, 174

F

Fallon, Joan, D.C., 71
FDA. *See* Food and Drug Administration.
Fischer, Martin, 41
Fisher, Barbara Loe, 13, 95
Flu, 90–97, 152–6
    avian, 152–6
    pandemics, 20-21, 48-57, 155–6

shots, 30–31, 52, 90-97
shots and Alzheimer's, 95
Spanish pandemic, 20-21
swine, 48–57
and Tamiflu, 52, 155
and Vitamin D, 93–94
Flu-Mist, 53
Fluoridation, 176–83
in California, 177, 179
and cavities, 176, 179, 182
chemicals in, 177
Fluoride, 178
Fluoride, 176-83
optimal amount, 181–2
sources of, 182
toxicity, 180
Food and Drug Administration
(FDA), 11–13, 22, 24–28, 30, 47,
64, 82, 87, 121, 122, 126, 127,
134, 136, 143, 145, 149, 158–60,
166-7, 181, 186, 189-90
Food and Nutrition Board, 196
Foods, and asthma, 137
and colds, 145
definition, 25-26
genetically modified, 4
nutritional quality of, 63–66
and viruses, 157–60
Franklin, Benjamin, 157, 205
Free-standing birth centers, 111
Fudenburg, Hugh, M.D., 95

G
Gardasil, 84, 87
Geison, Gerald, 35
Genes, 43–44
Genetically modified foods, 4
Germ theory, 34–37
Gerson, Max, M.D., xii
Glasser, George C., 178
Glavin, Margaret O'K., 12
Golomb, Beatrice, M.D., 129
Green, Alan, M.D., 140
Guide to Clinical Preventive Services, 81

H
H1N1. *See* swine flu.
Hanna, Cordelia S., 112
Harper, Diane, M.D., 85–86
Hartley, Carla, 114
Heard, George W., D.D.S., 179
Heart disease, 128-32, 205–9
Hepatitis B, 79-89
Herbert, Frank, 48
Hippocrates, 20, 21, 65, 68
Hirzy, J. William, Ph.D., 182
Hoffer, Abram, M.D., 64
Hoffman, Rita, 19
Holick, Michael F., M.D., Ph.D.,
196
Homeopath, 20, 21
Honaker, Richard, M.D., 196
Horne, Jim, Ph.D., 169
Hospital births, 107-14
Housman, Lawrence, 103
HPV, 79-89
Human Genome Project, 44
Huxley, Aldous, 139
Hygiene hypothesis, 38–42

I
Insomnia, 165–9
drugs for, 165-9
Institute of Medicine (IOM), 175,
195
International Cesarean Awareness
Network, 113
International Serious Adverse Event
Consortium (ISAEC), 47

J
Jamois, Tonya, 113
Jefferson, Tom, M.D., 57, 91
Jones, Glenville, Ph.D., 195–6
Journal of Applied Physiology, 68
Journal of Bone and Mineral Research,
181
Journal of Clinical Investigation, 76
Journal of Dental Research, 179

Journal of Human Hypertension, 99, 209
Journal of Manipulative and Physiological Therapeutics, 137
Journal of Orthomolecular Medicine, 66
Journal of the American Medical Association (JAMA), 47, 64–65, 69, 70, 150, 207
Journal of the Association of American Physicians and Surgeons, 31
Journal of the National Cancer Institute, 171

K
Kalokerinos, Archie, M.D., 78
Kazan, Elia, 49
Kennedy, John F., 73
Kieny, Dr. Marie Paul, 54
Kilpi, Dr. Terhi, 54
Kocher, Gerhard, 9
Kopel, Dave, 29

L
Lancet, 40, 178
Landon, Michael, 79
Langsjoen, Peter, M.D., 131
Leacock, Stephen, 161
Lee, John, M.D., 208
Lenzer, Jeanne, 85
Levine, Mark, M.D., 187
Levy, David, M.D., 11
Limeback, Hardy, Ph.D., D.D.S., 179
Lind, James, 65
Linkletter, Art, 203
Lipton, Bruce, Ph.D., 44-45
Living standards, 2

M
Magnesium, 189-93
Mammograms, 173–4
Marx, Groucho, 184
Maulik, Dev, 116

Mayo Clinic, 201
McBean, Eleanor, 88
McClenahan, John L., 147
McCormick, Dr. Marie, 54
McGinnis, J. Michael, Dr., 185
Measles, 9–17. *See also* vaccination.
Medical News Today, 134
Medline, 66
Medscape Today, 201
Mendelsohn, Robert S., M.D., xii, 15, 46–47
Merck & Co., 84
Microbes, 15, 34–37
Midwives, 105–6, 107–14
Migraines, 189-90
and magnesium, 191
Morning sickness, 103–6
Muldoon, Matthew, M.D., 130
Mumps, 15, 17. *See also* vaccination.

N
Nash, Ogden, 143
National Cancer Institute (NCI), 170–2
National Institute of Allergy and Infectious Disease, 53
National Institutes of Health (NIH), 66, 88, 169, 172, 184-7
National Poison Data System, 186
National Vaccine Information Center (NVIC), 83, 95
Naumann, Markus, M.D., 190
NCI. *See* National Cancer Institute.
Newborns, survival rate, 107
vaccination of, 80-84
New England Journal of Medicine, 11, 84, 112, 117, 171
New Scientist, 137
New York Daily News, *145*
New York Times, 131, 172
Null, Gary, Ph.D., 149

O
Obesity, 198–201

and chronic inflammation, 198–9, 201

factors in, 200

and health problems, 200

and NSAIDS, 201

surgical solutions, 201

Odent, Michael, M.D., 117

Oncologist, 171

Orenstein, Dr. Walter, 96

Orient, Jane, M.D., 83

Orthomolecular medicine, 66

news service, 195

treatment of disease, 67

Oski, Frand, M.D., 111

Osteopath, 20, 21

P

Palevsky, Lawrence B., M.D., 42, 95

Palmer, B. J., D.C., Ph.C., xi

Pap smears, 85-7, 121

Parapertussis, 74

Pasteur, Louis, 35–36

Pauling, Linus, Ph.D., 66

Pediatrics, 75, 199

Pertussis. *See* whooping cough.

Picoult, Jodi, 90

Pierce, Tanya Harter, 171

Placebo, 147-51

Plotnikoff, Greg, M.D., 196

Pollock, Channing, 58

Pregnancy, 2, 29–33, 103–6

and flu shots, 29-33, 53–54, 95

and midwives, 105–14

and ultrasounds, 115–119

Prehypertension, 121

Prescription drugs, 2-8, 22-23, 25-28, 47, 63, 69-70, 98-102, 123-7, 128-32, 133-8, 148-51, 161-4, 165-9, 185, 205-9

Primal Health Research Centre, 117

Proust, Marcel, 137

Psychology Today, 66

Public Health Policy Advisory Board, 134

Public Health Service, 181

Q

Quarterly Journal of the International Society for Fluoride Research, 178

R

Radiation, ultrasound, effects of, 116-17

x-ray, and increased breast cancer risk, 173-5

Rankin, Jeanette, 172

Rauch, Daniel, M.D., 145

Reason Magazine, 135

Recombivax HB, 82

Richwine, Lisa, 126–7

Rimland, Bernard, Ph.D., xii

Ritalin, 127

Robbins, John, 21

Rosch, Paul, M.D., 131

Rosedale, Don, M.D., 206, 207

Roses, Allen, M.D., 148, 149

Rousseau, Jean-Jacques, 202

Rush, Dr. Benjamin, 21

S

Santoli, Dr. Jeanne, 96

Saul, Andrew, Ph.D., 43

Schuchat, Anne, M.D., 55

Semmelweis, Ignaz Philip, xii

Seven laws for saving lives, 22–23

Sexually transmitted disease (STD), 79-89

Sharfstein, Joshua, M.D., 144-5

Shingles, 17

Simmons, Charles, 38

Simone, Charles B., Dr., 174

Sircus, Mark, Ac., O.M.D., 191

Sleep, 139–42

and ADHD, 140

and test scores, 140

Smith, Lendon, M.D., 125

Spina bifida, 30

Starfield, Barbara, M.D., Ph.D., 150

Start Later for Excellence in
Education Proposal (SLEEP), 142
Statins, 128–32, 205–8
side effects, 129-32, 206
STD. *See* sexually transmitted
disease.
Strand, Ray, 163
Surgeon General, 134
Suydam, Linda A., 143
Swine flu, 48–57, 155–6
Szent-Györgyi, Albert, 194

T
Tamiflu, 52, 155
Tamoxifen, 172
Tenpenny, Sheri, D.O., 81
Thermal imaging, 174
Thomas, Roger, Ph.D., M.D., 94
Tikkun Magazine, 173
Tom-Revzon, Katherine, 145
Toxins, 4–6, 60
Tritten, Jan, 109
Trust Birth, 114
Tuchman, Barbara, 170
Two-disease theory, 58–61

U
Ultrasound and pregnancy, 115–19
adverse effects of, 116
unneeded, 116, 118

V
Vaccination, 2-3, 5-7, 9–14, 17–19,
79–89
cervical cancer, 84–87
flu, 29-33, 48-57, 90–97, 152-6
hepatitis B, 80–84
HPV, 80, 84–87
investigating the need for, 84
MMR, 9-14
of newborns, 81
STD, 80
whooping cough, 73-78
Vaccine, 11, 32

Vaccine Adverse Event Reporting
System (VAERS), 54, 83, 86
Vaccines, and asthma, 137
disposal of, 96
and toxins, 5–6
Vaccine-induced disease, 83, 95, 137
Vaccine Information Awareness
Network, 19
Virginia Hopkins Health Watch
newsletter, 208
Viruses, 157–60
Vitamin D, 93-94, 194–7
recommended dosage, 196
Vitamin D Council, 93–94, 195
Vitamin supplements, 56, 64-67,
184–8, 194–7
Voltaire, 128
Von Tannenberg, Agnes Sallet, 107

W
Wagner, Marsden, 109
Wait-and-see prescription (WASP),
70
Wall Street Journal, 185
Washington Post, 143-5
WebMD, 99
Wellness, 63–68
Whitaker, Julian, M.D., 206-8
WHO. *See* World Health
Organization.
Whooping cough, 17, 73–78
deaths from, 74. *See also*
vaccination.
Wilk, Chester, D,C., 100
World Health Organization
(WHO), 33, 48–49, 75, 153-5

X
X rays, and cancer risk, 173-5

Y
Y2K, 153
Yazbak, F. Edward, M.D., 31, 83
Young, Jason, 124